The Blue Cotton Gown

The Blue Cotton Gown

A Midwife's Memoir

❈

Patricia Harman

BEACON PRESS, BOSTON

Beacon Press
25 Beacon Street
Boston, Massachusetts 02108–2892
www.beacon.org

Beacon Press books
are published under the auspices of
the Unitarian Universalist Association of Congregations.

13 12 11 10   8 7 6 5 4 3 2 1

This book is printed on acid-free paper that meets the uncoated paper
ANSI/NISO specifications for permanence as revised in 1992.

Text design and composition by Susan E. Kelly
at Wilsted & Taylor Publishing Services

Library of Congress Cataloging-in-Publication Data

Harman, Patricia
The blue cotton gown : a midwife's memoir / Patricia Harman.
p. ; cm.
ISBN 978-0-8070-7291-2 (alk. paper)
1. Harman, Patricia 2. Midwives—United States—Biography. I. Title.
[DNLM: 1. Harman, Patricia 2. Nurse Midwives—Personal Narratives.
3. Midwifery—Personal Narratives. WZ 100 H287 2008]

RG950.H36 2008
618.20092—dc22
[B]   2008007617

A portion of the first chapter originally appeared in the
Journal of Midwifery and Women's Health.

To midwife: To be with women, at childbirth and for life.

AUTHOR'S NOTE

The Blue Cotton Gown is based on my experiences and stories told to me by my patients. All names, identifiable characteristics, details of time, and names of places have been changed for the sake of preserving confidentiality. Several patients, professionals, and staff are composites. The events and conversations described are how I remember them.

Heartfelt thanks to every precious woman who has shared her story with me in her thin blue cotton exam gown, and to every health-care provider who has persisted in his or her calling despite personal and professional obstacles. We each have our own story. This is mine.

Patricia Harman, CNM

✳

Spring

CHAPTER I

Confessional

I have insomnia . . . and I drink a little. I might as well tell you. In the middle of the night, I drink scotch when I can't sleep. Actually, I can't sleep most nights; actually, every night. Even before I stopped delivering babies, I wanted to write about the women. Now I have time.

It's 2:00 a.m., and I pull my white terry bathrobe closer, thinking about the patients whose stories I hear. There's something about the exam room that's like a confessional. It's not dim and secret the way I imagine a confessional is in a Catholic church, the way I've seen them in movies. I peer at the clock. It's now 2:06.

The exam room where these stories are shared is brightly illuminated with recessed lighting. The walls are painted off-white and have a wallpaper border of soft leaves and berries. There are framed photographs of babies and flowers and trees, pictures I took myself and hung to make the space seem less clinical, and a bulletin board with handouts on stress reduction, wellness, and calcium.

The room is not big. It's the usual size. If I had to guess, I'd say eight feet by ten feet. The countertop under the tall white cupboard is hunter green, and there's a small stainless-steel sink in the corner. Other than a guest chair, my rolling stool, and a small trash can with a lid, there's just the exam table, angled away from the wall, with a flowered pillow and rose vinyl upholstery. On it lies a folded white sheet and a blue cotton gown with two strings for a tie. The exam table dominates everything.

I don't drink for fun. I don't even like scotch. It's for the sleep. I can't work if I can't sleep. The scotch is my sleep medicine and I want it to taste like medicine. The little jam jar with the black line at three ounces sits in the bathroom cupboard. My husband fills it for me, then locks the bottle in the closet. I ask him to do that. When you have as many alcoholics in your family as I do, you don't take chances. On nights when I'm restless, I drink it down sip by sip, making a bad face after each swallow. Then in an hour, I go back to bed.

I stand now at the window listening to the song of the spring frogs and thinking of the stories the women tell me, and then, in the stillest part of the deep night, I sit down to write. I need to sleep . . . but I need to tell the stories. The stories need to be told because they are from the hearts of women; the tender, angry hearts; the broken, beautiful hearts of women.

HEATHER

It's Monday morning and I'm late again. Waving to the receptionists, I rush through the waiting room. They turn to greet me in their aqua checked scrubs but keep on with their work. I know they keep track of how often I'm tardy.

"Hi, Donna," I say as I pull open the heavy cherry door to the clinical area. Donna, at the checkout desk, looks over her sleek horn-rim glasses and gives me a smile. The phone is tucked under her ear and she's clacking away at her computer.

Around the corner and down the hall is my office. It's small, just enough room for a desk, a file cabinet, two bookcases, and a guest chair. The cream walls are lined with my photographs: the highland forest in full autumn color, a pregnant woman stepping out of the shower, and our barn with the red roof next to our cottage in

Canada. On the window ledge are purple African violets rooted in a green pot that Tom threw on the wheel in his studio and a framed photo of the five of us last Christmas. I toss my briefcase into the corner.

In the picture, three mostly grown boys, Mica, Orion, and Zen, clown in front of the slightly crooked spruce tree. That's me in the back, with round pink cheeks, short straight brown hair streaked with gray, and wide blue eyes; a tall, girlish, middle-aged woman. Tom, stocky, slightly balding, with wire-rim glasses and short gray hair, stands with his arms around me. He's laughing too. It would take a miracle drug to get us all looking normal in front of a camera.

The Women's Health Clinic is located in Torrington, home of Torrington State University, on the fifth floor of the Family Health Center. Our private practice is composed of Tom Harman, ob-gyn; our two nurse-practitioners; and a staff of seven nurses and secretaries, all women. The suite, which we designed ourselves, is arranged in a rectangle with nine exam rooms, five offices, a lab, and a conference room. There's also a small kitchen, the waiting room, and the large secretaries' area up front. On two sides, windows run the length of the office. I wanted the staff and the patients to be able to look out at the sky.

Five minutes after I arrive, I'm standing in the exam room holding out my hand to a skinny young woman who stares at it as if she's just been offered something she'd rather not touch, a dead fish or rotten banana. She has short curly red hair, a beautiful girl, but she holds her head down like she doesn't know it. An eyebrow ring mars her perfect face. I pull my hand back and try again. "I'm Patsy Harman, nurse-midwife, you must be . . ."—glancing at the new chart—"Heather Moffett."

Heather doesn't say hello or anything else. There's also an older woman and a young man in the room, so I start talking to them, turning first to the older lady who's sitting in the guest chair, clutching her large white pocketbook. "And you are . . . family?" The grim-faced, gray-haired woman nods once. She inspects me through her glasses, clear plastic frames with rhinestones at the corners.

I was hoping she would introduce herself. "Heather's mother or aunt . . . ?" I prompt. It's always better to flatter than insult, though the woman appears to be in her seventies.

"I'm her grandma."

This is not a cordial group, and I'm wondering what kind of con-versation they were having before I came in. The air feels like ce-ment just beginning to harden. "And you?" I turn to the young man.

"T.J.," he responds sullenly. That's all he says.

Heather is sitting hunched over on the small built-in bench in the dressing corner of the exam room, her arms tucked into her blue exam gown. T.J. swivels back and forth on my stool. The grand-mother is perched on the one gray guest chair, so there's nowhere left for me to sit except the exam table, and that isn't going to happen.

"Before we get started, let's rearrange things," I say energetically. "Heather, you sit up here on the exam table. T.J., you sit where she was, and I'll take the stool." We all trade places and when the young man stands I realize he's over six feet tall. His hair reaches past his shoulders and he's good-looking, like a heavy-metal star in the eight-ies, thin and sensuous with flat gray-blue eyes. No one says any-thing. They just move to where I point.

"So." I start up once more. "It looks like you're going to have a baby, Heather. Were you trying, or did it just happen?" I ask it like this, not wanting to assume every teenage pregnancy is an accident. Heather shrugs and glances at T.J.

I try again. "So are you excited, or still in shock?"

"Excited, I guess," Heather says, not sounding like she is.

"Well, that's nice, then," I respond. The grandmother rolls her pale, watery blue eyes and crosses her ankles, which look purple and sore.

"Let me go over what you've written in your history, and then I'll ask you more questions. Today what we need to do is an exam and some lab work—" I don't get to finish.

"I got to puke," says Heather, standing up with her hand over her mouth and searching wildly around. The grandmother and I stand up too. The older woman opens her bag and comes up with some tissues. I take Heather's slender arm and lead her to the small stainless-steel sink. T.J. stays where he is. This doesn't involve him. Heather gags.

"Do you have time to get to the bathroom?" I ask. The patient stands still, her head down, her red hair hanging around her face. I pull the curls back, holding them out of the way. Nothing comes up.

"I'm okay . . . I think," Heather whispers.

"Has she been vomiting a lot, Mrs. . . . ?"

"It's Gresko, Mrs. Gresko. A fair 'mount, yes. Three, four times a day, seems like, maybe more."

I take the girl's pulse. It's rapid, and when I pinch the pale skin on her forearm, it tents, a sign of dehydration. "Are you keeping *anytl.ing* down?"

"Some," says the grandmother. "She's bleeding too." Our eyes meet, and when I look over, I see blood dripping down Heather's legs.

"When did this start?"

"Yesterday. That's why we called 'round for an appointment. I don't want nothin' to happen to this baby."

So much for taking a detailed, organized history. "You know, Heather, I've changed my mind. I'll read what you wrote on the OB form and ask you questions next visit. Since you're feeling so sick, I'd just like to get you a prescription for the vomiting and—"

"What about the blood?" T.J. challenges. "That isn't good, is it?"

"No, it isn't. It isn't a good sign, but it doesn't always mean something bad. How much blood is there?"

Heather looks at her grandmother.

"'Bout like her monthly," Mrs. Gresko says.

"Can you tell me when your last real period was?"

Heather shrugs.

"We can't be sure," says Grandma. "I tell her to write down her *time* but she don't."

Great, I think. "Well, why don't you lie back on the exam table and I'll feel your belly to see if I can get an idea." My hands palpate Heather's lower abdomen. There's a bulge halfway between her jeweled belly-button ring and the pubic bone, about right for fourteen weeks. Could the girl really be that far along?

"Give me a minute. I want to see if my husband, Dr. Harman, is available for an ultrasound." I leave, shaking my head, and trot down the hall. Looking through the window in the nurses' station, I see storm clouds have come in from the west.

Tom's two exam rooms are on the opposite side of the clinic, and both doors are closed, indicating there are patients inside. Behind one, I can hear voices, and I knock softly, nervous about interrupting him.

No one answers, and I tap again, louder, hoping he's not in the middle of a pelvic exam. Finally he opens the door. "What's up?" He's wearing a red checked shirt with a Beatles tie and black Dockers. His white lab coat is reserved for the hospital. He would wear jeans and a corduroy shirt to the office if I let him.

"I have a new OB that's spotting; can you do an ultrasound for viability and dating?" I ask. "Do you have time?"

Tom glances at his watch and shakes his head. "I have three patients to see before I go to the OR. Is she bleeding heavily? Can we do it tomorrow?"

I shrug. "It's not like she's hemorrhaging. But it's not good either, and they're anxious."

"Get her here in the morning, I'll squeeze her in." A middle-aged woman sitting on the exam table glares at me through aviator glasses. Tom closes the door, and I head down the hall, trying to decide what to say.

I could scan Heather myself, but even if I can find the heartbeat she'll need a second ultrasound to get an accurate gestational age. And if it *is* a miscarriage, I want Tom to be there to confirm it. The family won't like having to return, but tomorrow is best.

When I reenter the exam room I find the small group standing in a knot next to the sink. They quickly sit down. "She *threw up*," says Mrs. Gresko, as if it's my fault.

"What about the ultrasound?" demands T.J.

"I'm sorry," whispers the girl, looking down.

I go to the sink. They've cleaned it, but it still smells like vomit. The nurses will have to spray with disinfectant. "We'll have to do the ultrasound tomorrow. I'm sorry. If the bleeding gets worse tonight, come to the ER. I know you're worried, but you have to understand that if a miscarriage is going to happen, nothing can stop it. Just rest, get some ginger ale for hydration, and come in around ten. I'll write you a script for medicine that might help with the nausea, and you could try some peppermint tea. I have a feeling everything's going to be all right . . ." I'm not sure why I say this.

Mrs. Gresko shifts in her seat and sighs with irritation. T.J. crosses his long legs in disgust. Heather studies her stubby blue fingernails.

So far she's uttered all of four sentences, and that's all I'm going to get.

Blood

When I got up to pee in the white enamel commode, it was dark and I couldn't see the blood dripping down my legs. I didn't bother to light the kerosene lamp. This was downstairs in the log cabin, back in the commune days.

Because my first pregnancy with Mica had gone without a hitch, miscarriage was the last thing I had on my mind. When I saw the brown streak in my underwear that morning, I didn't even know what it was. It didn't occur to me that the streak was old blood, and I didn't bother to call my doctor. Then again, I couldn't have, since we didn't have a phone; not that there was anything a doctor could have done anyway.

By afternoon I began to bleed in earnest. I wasn't a midwife yet, but I understood. Tom and I cried together. In the night, the fire in the woodstove went out, but we had thick quilts and were used to the cold.

Most women don't have more than menstrual cramps when they miscarry, but for me the pain came like labor contractions. If I could have gotten up and walked around, it would have been easier. I might have built up the fire or asked my husband to, but I just stayed under the covers.

With a towel between my legs, I lay doing my childbirth breathing. Mica slept curled in his little homemade bed across the room. Tom adjusted the pillow under his bad shoulder. He knew what was happening but he wasn't a physician then, hadn't even thought of becoming one. He asked if I needed anything. I didn't. What could he do?

When I got up at dawn I was dizzy. In the gray light I saw the sheets covered in red. I lay back down in the warm blood and stared out the window. During the night, it had snowed. The oaks and maples on our West Virginia ridge were covered in white; the pine trees, the cedars, everything.

NILA

Nila speaks first. "So, I guess you're surprised to see me." The five-foot-tall dishwater blonde leans back on the exam table, swinging her bare legs like a girl. The blue cotton exam gown is three sizes too big.

"No, not surprised to see you, just surprised to see you *pregnant*. I thought Gibby was going to get a vasectomy. Did he change his mind?"

"Nah, he never got it." Nila pauses. "I've been living in Independence, South Dakota, for over a year."

"Did the receptionist tell you we stopped delivering babies?"

"That's what I heard; they said you gave up births a few months ago, but I don't have any money and I haven't been to the health department to get a medical card. I figured you'd see me anyway."

She gives me a smile, and she's right. At our clinic, we see new OBs even if they aren't established patients, regardless of payer status. We try to help them get medical cards, back-billing if they qualify, setting up payment plans if they don't. Tom and I were poorer than poor when we lived on the farm. We know how it is.

"It was the cost of malpractice insurance. Last year the practice premiums for obstetrics went from seventy thousand dollars a year to a hundred and ten thousand. We just couldn't do it. *A hundred and ten thousand a year!* You could buy a pretty good house in West Virginia for a hundred and ten thousand dollars, a new one every twelve months." The patient nods sympathetically. I tell all the new OB patients why we gave up deliveries. I give them the numbers, hoping they'll understand.

Nila is a "grand multip," meaning she's had more than five babies. In all her pregnancies she's never had a miscarriage, a C-section, or a stillbirth. She smokes, has poor nutrition, and when not pregnant weighs about a hundred pounds. I delivered babies five, six, and seven. Most people think the more babies a mother has, the easier it gets, but that's not true. After baby five, it gets harder. By that time, the uterus is so stretched, it doesn't contract well. Malpresentations (breech, transverse, face), prolonged labor, and hemorrhage are common. Nila's seventh one was the worst.

I can still see Nila lying in the birthing bed, thin, flat-chested, with smooth tan skin. She has the high cheekbones and small chin of a lot of Appalachian women, and when she smiles, her two front teeth gap a little, but not badly. The petite thirty-eight-year-old was fully dilated, her epidural topped off, and she was as comfortable as a breast-fed baby, but she wouldn't push.

"Come on, Nila," I pleaded. "Come on. You can do it! Two or three more pushes and it'll all be over. *Then* you can rest."

"I'm tired; I want to rest *now.*"

Nila's labor had been long. It started at two in the morning. At four in the afternoon, she'd been given Phenergan IV for her nausea.

❄   ❄   ❄

Now sunset, the baby is poised at the opening of the vagina, ready to be born, but the mother's half drunk from the medicine and won't cooperate.

"*Please,* Nila. Just grab my hand and push hard." I nod at her husband, Gibby, indicating *he* should say something.

"Yeah, come on, honey . . ." Not much enthusiasm. He's tired too.

The RN catches my eye and turns up the volume on the fetal heart monitor. *Beep . . . beep . . . . beep . . . . beep . . . . beep.* The fetal heart rate is dipping with each contraction. This baby needs to be born.

Nila closes her eyes, as if she actually thinks we might let her nap, then coughs. It's a raspy deep smoker's cough, and with the abdominal effort the baby's dark hairy head moves down an inch. "Hey, do that again."

"What?" Nila asks, her eyes still shut.

"Cough. Cough again. It's moving the baby."

The patient rouses. "Like that?" She coughs again and the fetal head pokes out a little more. I glance at the monitor. Heart rate to seventy, but back to 120 by the end of the contraction.

"Yeah, keep going. You might be my first patient to *cough* her baby out." Nila giggles, forces another cough, and laughs at herself.

The rhythmic shaking of her belly works even better than the cough, and the baby's head shows some more.

"Look," says the nurse, pulling over a mirror on a wheeled stand. "You can see your baby being born." Now we are all getting into it, telling Nila we'll tickle her and offering knock-knock jokes. Even Gibby participates, whispering something into his wife's ear that makes her blush and giggle some more.

I place my hands around the baby's emerging head like a crown, easing back the perineum. The nurse slips me warm compresses and oil to help the skin stretch, and a small vigorous baby slips into my hands.

"Gonna call him the Joker," Gibby quips as the nurse places the wailing pink infant into his arms. Nila has already fallen asleep . . .

❧   ❧   ❧

I smile now, remembering . . . then shake my head and return to the exam room.

"So you and Gibby moved west. Did he get work there?"

"No, I went by myself, just me and the kids. All but the oldest, who's a senior in high school. He wanted to stay in Torrington to graduate. After the accident, Gibby wasn't quite right. He took it out on me. So one day I just loaded up and moved out."

My mind's reeling. First, I can't remember what accident she's talking about. Had it been before or after the last birth? Second, how many kids in a car would that be?

"He took it out on you? You mean, hit you?"

"No, not really hit, but it was going that way. Pushed me around, just a few bruises and one time a burn."

"So you just left?"

"Yeah, I planned it all out. I waited until he'd left for work. He was gone by six. I was packed and loaded by six thirty, then I woke up the kids."

I can see Nila bustling around getting the six children dressed, her short brown-blond hair whipping as she works. *No school today,* she says cheerfully. *We're going on a trip, an overnight. A big adventure.*

Where? Where? the little kids say.

What about my baseball tonight? What about my slumber party? the middle ones ask.

The oldest daughter tries to get the kids into their jackets. She doesn't complain. She knows her mom needs her.

At last they pile into the van. It would have to be a van, with that many kids. Nila passes out the juice boxes and the Pop-Tarts for breakfast, and they shut up. She turns on some oldies rock music on the radio and pulls out of the drive. The sun's just rising over the mountains.

"You just left?" I ask now. "You took the kids and went to South Dakota? Did you know someone there?"

"No, I just drove and drove, and when I got to Independence, it was a smallish town and seemed like a nice place to raise children, so I stayed."

"But how did you live?" I ask, amazed. "Did you find work?"

"I had a few hundred dollars saved, and then Gibby had to send money."

I squint, trying to understand. "Did you sort of run away from home?"

"You could *say* that." Nila laughs. "Well, I met a fella out there, his name's Doug and he was real nice to me, and here I am." She pats her belly, which is already rounding. So it's not Gibby's baby. She doesn't seem upset. In fact, she seems happy. I'm still pondering the overwhelming prospect of getting in a car with that many kids and just hitting the road.

"Do you have a place to live? Did Gibby take you back?" If he had taken her back when she was pregnant by another man, that would be as amazing as Nila's packing up and leaving home in the first place!

"Oh, no. Doug and I found an old farmhouse out on Weimer Road."

"Doug came back with you and all the kids? Did you *mean* to have his baby?"

"Well, not right away, but we thought maybe later."

I frown. "Were you using any birth control, pills or condoms?"

"No, not really." Nila giggles and rolls her eyes.

"So, has Doug found a job?"

"Oh, yeah, right away, at Select-Tech, that telemarketing place downtown." Nila smiles proudly.

"But what about your husband? How's he handling this?" I picture the quiet blond man who had come to Nila's births. He's employed in maintenance for one of the big student-housing companies in Torrington.

"Oh, Gibby's acting like a jerk, keeps coming over or trying to call me. If Doug's home and answers, he hangs up . . . I shouldn't have expected him to be decent. I have to let him see the kids, though. Unless he's drinking. If I smell alcohol on his breath, he's out of there."

I warm up my hands by rubbing them together and motion for Nila to lie back on the exam table. Her uterus is easily palpable under my fingers. "Have you felt movement yet? It's probably too early."

"No, I feel it. Not every day, but I feel it." She smiles at the ceiling. "After seven kids, you know that the baby is in there."

There are red flags waving, but I don't see them. I'm worried about how late I'm running and how many other women are waiting in the reception area. I'm thinking about all my patients who feel trapped by unhealthy relationships, financial burdens, or family troubles, women with many more resources than Nila but not a bit of her courage. They come into the office year after year, enduring the same old things, taking Paxil or Prozac so they can cope.

"So why'd you come back?"

"I missed the Green Mountains. I just missed them."

HEATHER

At 10:15 a.m., Heather Moffett and her family return and are escorted to the ultrasound room. The little group shuffles past my office door and heads down the long hall. Today Mrs. Gresko is dressed in a long navy-dotted shirtwaist. She stops to straighten a framed photograph of a lone oak tree on the wall as she passes.

I wait for them to get settled, staring out the window at the gray sky for a few minutes. I saw trillium blooming this morning on my way to work, white bells at the edge of the forest. Outside, the sun goes in and out of the clouds.

This morning Tom's ultrasound room is crowded. T.J. sits in the only chair available, and Mrs. Gresko stands, still clutching her white purse. Heather lies passively on her back with her legs bent; a white half-sheet is over her lap, and she's wearing a skimpy pink T-shirt. The large ultrasound machine stands in the corner, a printer beside it. The family smells strongly of cigarettes.

Dr. Harman has already started. His RN, Sherry—black shiny hair cut short in a bob, always pleasant, the archetypal nurse—stands ready to assist. "If the baby's too early we may not see a heartbeat yet," Tom is explaining. He adjusts a few knobs. Today he wears his tan Dockers and a pale blue dress shirt. A stethoscope hangs around his neck. His close-cut gray hair needs a trim.

"By my exam," I interject, "Heather feels about fourteen weeks pregnant, but she can't remember her last period, so we're not sure how far along she is, and there's been some spotting."

Tom is silent. He's in a get-it-done mood, no chitchat. As he does the internal vaginal ultrasound, he uses his more sensitive right hand to palpate the abdomen. Then he presses a few more buttons on the console. A tiny fetus resembling a tadpole comes into view. I expected it to be bigger.

Dr. Harman points out the baby. I always call Tom "Doctor" when we're with patients. It's a formal convention, a way of reminding myself that our relationship in the clinic and the hospital is professional. I motion T.J. to come closer. Despite the young man's reserve, he stands up. "There it is!" I whisper. "There's the heartbeat." I squeeze Heather's gaunt arm. She's so thin, it crosses my mind that she could be anorexic. No one seems as excited as I am, but the tension drops in the room. Despite the spotting, the baby's still alive. It's always a thrill to see that heart beating.

"It's about seven weeks, and has a good pulse," Dr. Harman informs the group, printing out a picture. He hands it to Heather. "There's your baby." He grins. I like that smile, wide with straight teeth. Heather and her grandma inspect the small photograph. T.J. glances down but doesn't move closer. The screen swirls as Tom inspects the patient's ovaries. He's surveying for cysts or any other abnormality.

"Looks pretty good," he says. "You can turn the lights up." He nods to me and I reach for the rheostat. "Wait," he says, inspecting the screen intently, moving the vaginal transducer from side to side. I dim the lights again and the mood dims as well, each of us wondering what could be wrong.

"There's another one," Tom announces. Two tiny fetuses lie side by side. Heather looks at me.

"There are *two* babies. Two heartbeats. You have twins!" I tell her, understanding now why my estimate of her dates was so wrong. "No wonder you've been so sick." The girl smiles for the first time, and her thin pixie face lights up. She glances at T.J., who stands just a little taller. On the other hand, Grandma tightens her square jaw and looks away. She knows how hard it is to take care of one baby, let alone two.

By the time Heather gets to the checkout desk, everyone in the office, from RN to billing specialist, knows the young woman is having twins. The staff gathers to congratulate the family. Sometimes I think that they miss the thrill of doing deliveries more than I do.

It's odd how excited people get about twins. In my mind, it's double trouble, a difficult pregnancy with preterm labor and maybe preeclampsia. And a potentially difficult delivery, with cord entanglement or fetal malpresentation.

Before the family leaves, I give them a packet of OB handouts and a lab-requisition slip. I manage to explain that we no longer deliver babies because of the high cost of medical-liability insurance. Heather seems disappointed. T.J. is mad, Grandma exasperated. "So who will she go to?" Mrs. Gresko demands.

"We can take care of Heather until she gets through the first three or four months. That will be three more visits. When we get her labs back and know the pregnancy is stable, I'll sit down with you and go over the options. There aren't as many choices in OB providers as there used to be, but I can find someone you'll like. Try not to worry too much about the bleeding. There's a good chance it will stop."

It occurs to me that Heather may not have insurance, and a glance at the front of the chart confirms it. SELF-PAY, the sticker reads. "Have you applied for a medical card yet?" I ask quietly.

"We will," Mrs. Gresko says firmly. At least she's aware of the financial reality. I'm just hoping that Heather will qualify. If a woman is poor enough, there isn't a problem. It's the folks slightly above that line who get screwed, the working poor and the self-employed. If you're living on minimum wage, there's no way you can pay seven hundred dollars for a family health-care policy.

There's so much I've not had time to talk to the girl about. Carrying twins changes everything. There will be an increased need for nutrition, increased need for rest. I write on the checkout slip for Heather to return in two weeks so I can finish her new-OB exam and we can talk more. Then, as we stand in the reception area, I manage to whisper in the girl's ear that she and T.J. shouldn't have intercourse until after the bleeding has stopped for ten days.

Heather gazes at me as if that's the last thing in the world a teenager would do.

HOLLY

Holly Knight, an attractive forty-five-year-old, is examining her manicured nails. "It's okay if you don't want to talk about it," I say. The exam room is quiet. There are no clocks ticking, except in my mind. I'm already half an hour behind schedule.

The prominent Torrington real estate agent is here for her annual exam. She's taller than I am, almost six feet, with broad shoulders. Since I'm tall myself, I notice these things. Her angular jaw and long limbs speak of a former athlete, maybe a tennis player. "It's okay if you don't want to talk about this," I repeat. I had asked her about her stress level.

Finally, Holly clears her throat, straightens her blue exam gown, and adjusts the silver clip that holds back her shoulder-length, highlighted hair. "It's my oldest daughter. She's just a beautiful girl. She *was* beautiful. Now she's in intensive care at a hospital in Charleston and looks like a skeleton. She has an eating disorder . . . I've never told anyone about this. If women ask at church or at the country club, I just say she has severe colitis."

I wait, imagining the young woman, a shadow of Holly, her translucent skin just covering the blue life pumping within her, propped up in a white hospital bed. There's a tube in her nose, IVs in both arms, and a heart monitor beeping away at the bedside, all that connects her to life.

The patient looks down, and the mask falls away. "Nora was so bright and lively and involved when she was in high school. She was in soccer, in debate club, in the school plays. I don't know how this happened. It must be my fault. She never seemed to have any weight problems when she was a kid. She would eat a good dinner. We even drank whole milk then." Holly looks up at me. Her green eyes are brimming. "I've thought about this a lot. Now I realize she was vomiting everything up. Now she can't stop vomiting. It must be my fault, but I don't know what I did.

"Think about it." She snorts a short laugh and with the tips of her fingers wipes her eyes. "Anyone who can drink that much whole milk and not gain weight has a problem, but I didn't see it. Maybe you only see what you want to."

I listen spellbound as the patient tells her story. I'm seeing myself only a few years ago, so alone with my troubles, embarrassed to tell anyone, a seemingly successful woman, sturdy, competent . . . crumbling inside. Holly continues, "I'm just so worried. I'm terrified she's going to die. Maybe this time or next time she'll die. We've been to counselors and clinics." She looks around as if she's lost her place in the story, but she hasn't. "This is the third time she's been hospitalized this year."

I say nothing. It isn't a therapeutic silence. I just can't think what to say.

There's a scratch at the door. It's my nurse Abby, alerting me patients are waiting. I glance at my watch and shake my head. I'm absorbed in this woman's pain and I know why. Once, I, too, had had no one to confide in, no friend or colleague whose children had been busted for grass, or for scrawling graffiti on the undersides of bridges, or for driving with an open bottle of alcohol.

I'm now an hour behind, but in the next five minutes I finish Holly's exam, write her a script for her antidepressant, and give her a handout on calcium. Then I sit again on my gray rolling stool, unsure how to end the encounter. Holly breaks the silence.

"Thank you for listening. I've never confessed this to anyone. No one knows but my husband and our three boys." She clears her throat. "We should have seen it coming. We should have gotten help sooner . . . I recognize it now."

When I stand, I don't know my intention. I could give the woman a hug. That's what I usually do, but instead I take Holly's head between my hands and press my forehead against hers, my straight short gray-brown hair against the silky waves. I'm surprised and not sure what I mean by this gesture, what I'm trying to tell her, but I stand there for a moment, the silence in my brain going into hers. She smells like roses. It hurts to be a mother. It hurts to give birth. And it can hurt a lot worse later.

Then I start to leave but pause at the door. "What did you say her name was? Your daughter?"

"It's Nora."

"I'll say a prayer for her," I whisper. Holly's eyes meet mine. "I'll say a prayer for her."

Prayer

There aren't many words to my prayers. I have a little box on our dresser. It's a round red wooden box, with a yellow moon and stars on the lid. I can't remember where it came from, probably a present from one of the boys.

Nora, Holly's daughter. May she eat and enjoy life and love herself, I write on a tiny slip of paper. And on another, *Holly, mother of Nora, may she forgive herself and find peace.* I open the box and gaze at the multicolored folded squares. There's a prayer for my brother Darren, crippled after a surgery and living in Texas. There are prayers for each of my sons, Mica, Orion, and Zen. And for Maria, who has breast cancer. And for Ruth, whose daughter was killed in an auto accident. I refold the prayers. The box is getting full, but I'm superstitious. If I take someone's prayer out too early, something bad might happen.

In my first years of nurse-midwifery school, I was taught not to mix religion with medicine. It wasn't considered professional, but lately I've broken the rule. I used to pray on my knees for the boys, passionately calling out for someone to hear. "*Please,* keep my boys out of trouble. Help them learn to walk away from danger. Give them some sense. Shine your light on them." I prayed the same words over and over every night. After a while, I realized I was badg-ering God. The Great Spirit had heard me the first time. I was prob-ably getting on his or her nerves.

Now, each night I light a small white candle. I put my hand on the round red box. "God be with you," I say, and my love goes into the air with the light, to my patients, my kids, whoever's in trouble. I don't know if it helps. It's my prayer.

One name I finally took out of the box is Lyndie. Lyndie died of breast cancer. I took her prayer out after the funeral.

One name I haven't put in is my own.

CHAPTER 2

Sin of Omission

"Didn't you notice?" Rebecca had asked, scratching her head with a pencil. "Didn't you check his figures?" Her red hair flared around her face, and her dangling earrings shimmered.

Now I turn over and pull the covers up to my chin, remembering the meeting with our new accountant from Pittsburgh. It's 2:15 a.m. and I need to sleep, but I can't. Rebecca Gorham had reviewed the letter we received from the IRS and told us that the practice owed the government twenty-one thousand dollars. The best I can understand is that our former accountant, Bob Reed, had been underreporting the corporate income for two years. "Didn't you check his figures?" Rebecca had asked again in frustration.

"No," answered Tom, pushing his wire-rim glasses up on his nose. "We trusted the man. It's his job. He knows about numbers, I know about medicine. If I checked everything he did, I might as well be my own accountant!"

Gorham had tossed her head, and her earrings had tinkled. "You understand that you're responsible for everything you sign, don't you? Your signature is on the tax returns; you'll be personally liable."

It's 2:25 a.m. I throw the covers back and crawl out of bed. In the bathroom I find my jam jar of scotch and pull my robe closer around me. I pad though the dark living room, moving by feel, past the sofa and love seat, dragging my fingers along the muted southwestern cream and blue upholstery. It's the same Pine Factory furniture we bought when Tom was an ob-gyn resident. The cream Berber carpet is soft under my feet.

In the corner, in front of four tall windows, a ten-foot ficus tree grows in a pot. If it weren't for the cathedral ceiling, there'd be nowhere to put it. I stand for a moment looking out, and then step through the glass door onto the wraparound porch. No peepers tonight. No stars.

This house, cedar sided, perches over Hope Lake. To the south, through the bare trunks of oaks, the water picks up light from cottages. Steep wooden steps lead down to the dock. I pace around the porch to the west.

Here two acres of grass spread gently uphill. In the moonlight I can dimly see Tom's beehives, our oval vegetable garden, and beyond that the gazebo. When we first moved to Blue Rock Estates, the yard was just mud. Now there are peach, pear, and apple trees and a few pines.

There's something about Rebecca that makes me uneasy. We've only been with her three months. Our failure with the previous accountant causes me to doubt my judgment. We've started with her now, so we'll continue. Tom trusts everyone, and he hates change. I don't much like it myself.

I take my first sip and swallow it down. The first sip is the worst . . . bitter and burning. There's no movement down at the lake, no sound, only the little waves lapping.

Rebecca has promised she'll contact the IRS and request an explanation of the bill. She'll argue that the error in underpayment, if there is one, was an oversight of the previous accountant and apply for an extension to give us some time. We've never owed money like this before, and I don't have a clue where we'll get it.

I gaze at the half-moon as it slips back and forth between the clouds, an unhappy lady, then I say a small prayer. Twenty-one thousand dollars!

TRISH

"What's wrong?" Trish catches my arm as I hurry out of the medical center and across the parking lot on my way to the car. I'm not sure I want to see her. Since the meeting with Rebecca Gorham, I've been walking around like a whipped dog. "You look awful. Are you getting sick?"

Trish is a nursing assistant in the Family Wellness office, two floors below the Torrington Women's Health Clinic. We've been friends for ten years, maybe twelve. Tom delivered her third baby and did her surgery when she had an ectopic pregnancy. She left the university medical practice to join Dr. Wilson at Community Hospital about the same time we left the faculty ob-gyn practice to start out on our own.

"I'm having a meltdown," I say grimly. Trish follows me to my car; her straight, cropped sandy blond hair blows across her face as she hauls her heavy satchel over her shoulder. I fumble with my keys at the Honda. "I feel like crying all the time."

"What? What's up? I've never seen you like this."

I get in the car, take a deep breath, and rub my hand over my face as I settle behind the steering wheel. "It's the IRS . . . We're screwed. We thought our first accountant, Bob Reed, was fine, but what did we know? I mean, Tom and I can barely balance a checkbook. Not that we *can't,* we just don't get around to it, know what I mean? Anyway, to make a long story short, the guy wasn't doing his job. We got a letter a few days ago saying we owe the Feds twenty-one thousand dollars!"

I let that sink in. Trish gets in the car, settles herself in the passenger seat, and pulls a pack of cigarettes out of her bag. Then, realizing we're sitting in my vehicle, not hers, she puts it back with a sheepish grin.

"Our new accountant, Rebecca, says it looks serious. And we don't have it, Trish! We don't have that kind of money, not in the practice and not at home. Tom and I just live month to month. We're paying off his student loans and the kids are still in college. We've never had much of a savings account and we're up to our ears in debt. I know if you walk into our office we look successful—nice furniture, nice carpet, and new equipment—but since Dr. Burrows left and took all his patients, it's been really tight. If this IRS thing is real, we could be ruined. I feel like such a screwup . . . Don't tell anyone, okay?"

My friend nods but is silent, then finally says, "Maybe it's a mistake."

"Yeah, we're praying."

"You'll work it out."

"Think so?"

Trish smiles, then reaches into the depths of her quilted flowered bag and pulls out a red tin. "*Know* so! Want a homemade chocolate chip cookie? It's better than tobacco. A patient brought them to the office, and my boss told me to take them home. The kids will never know what they're missing." Trish has a boy and two girls, Artie, Jennifer, and the oldest one, Aran.

"You know how to cheer a girl up." We sit, munching. I sigh. "I've been trying to cut out sweets, but there's a time and place for everything. Chocolate's a blessing, almost as good as an antidepressant." Trish shrugs. My friend is a perfect size 10 and never has to watch her weight. It might be because she smokes cigarettes. Whatever it is, I'm jealous.

Trish puts her hand over mine. "You'll work it out," she says again, glancing at the clock on the dashboard and gathering up her things. "*I've got to run!* I'm meeting Aran at the mall to shop for her prom dress. Can you believe she's graduating from high school in a few months? I'm only thirty-five, and my baby is graduating." I picture the slim teenager, so like her mother, same sandy hair, same blue eyes, only taller.

"Who's her date?"

"This kid Jimmy. He's from Pittsburgh. Dan doesn't like him. Thinks he's on drugs. Aran says she's *in love*. Do kids really know at that age? I tried to tell Dan that *my* parents didn't like *him* when we were seventeen either, thought he'd end up a bum, but we've done okay, been together almost twenty years."

I picture Dan, a tall, sweet guy who works as a tree trimmer for the state highway department.

"Got to rush!" She slams the Civic door and waves back to me.

When Dr. Harman was twenty and a bearded hippie, no one thought he would amount to anything either. "Hey, your cookies!" I yell through the open window, holding out the red tin.

"They're your cookies now!" Trish yells back.

REBBA

"My boyfriend told me I should ask you," the twenty-six-year-old starts out. "He thinks there might be something wrong with me. I might be frigid." I glance up from her chart. I've been seeing Rebba for three years, and this is the first time the young woman has mentioned sexual difficulties.

"Why would you say that?" I ask.

"Well, *you know*," Rebba says, "I don't find enjoyment like other women, and I've been with my fiancé for over a year. I've been with other men too. It just never happens."

"Do you get excited?" I scoot the exam stool up against the white wall so I can lean back.

Rebba nods. I watch her face. She has a flawless olive complexion. Her nose is narrow and straight. Long auburn hair.

"Do you have an orgasm?"

Rebba shrugs. "I don't know. Maybe . . . I like your gowns."

"What?"

"I like these exam gowns. My other doctor had paper ones. They gave me the creeps. Sometimes they'd tear, and they stood out like a paper lantern all around so you felt more naked under them than if you had nothing on. These are nice." She strokes the worn fabric.

I stare at the gown, frowning. It's plain pale blue print with tiny darker blue diamonds, nothing fancy, the usual hospital type. There's a tie at the neck. The utilitarian garment only comes in two sizes, large and extra large. That means it looks awful on everyone.

Even before we started our practice, I decided that the gowns had to be soft cotton to cover the delicate nakedness of our patients. "We rent them from the Mountain View Laundry so there's no choice of style. Thanks for noticing. They cost more, but it's worth it." I grin. "You're worth it." There's a pause while I try to find the tangled thread of the conversation. "You were saying . . . you aren't sure if you have an orgasm?" Rebba shrugs. "Do you know what they feel like?" She shrugs again. "An orgasm can be anything from a pleasant twitching in the vagina to something more like a whole body seizure with complete exhaustion afterward. Does any of this sound familiar?"

Rebba shakes her head, puzzled.

I try again. "Do you *want* to make love? Are you *in love* with your fiancé? Do you know what I mean, like desire him, want to kiss him?"

Rebba brightens and her eyes shine. "Oh, yeah, he's the best." Her face is flushed just talking about it. "That's why I had to ask you. I'm afraid he'll get tired of me if I don't . . . you know . . . learn to *come*. Do you have medicines or anything?" She trails off. There are tears in her eyes.

"Rebba," I say. "It may not be that important. I talk to lots of women. Many don't have orgasms but have happy lives. It may not be that important to everyone."

"*But it is to me,*" the girl whispers.

"I know what you mean." I let out a breath. "For me it is too. Let me ask you this: Do you ever feel frustrated *after* intercourse? Like you aren't finished and want to do more?"

The patient's hazel eyes lose focus as she tries to remember. "No, I guess I'm *relieved* when it's over, because if he goes on too long it hurts . . . Sometimes I wish he'd keep going with his mouth though."

This catches my attention. "Why does he stop?"

"I guess he gets bored. I never asked him."

"Did you tell him to keep going?"

"*No!*" Rebba's voice goes up, horrified, and she flashes a look at the ceiling.

"Why not?"

The young woman shakes her head. "Well, I'm *wet* then. He says that means I'm ready."

I sigh. It's time for the Chat. "Okay, Rebba, there are some things I think you and your partner don't quite understand." I wheel my stool closer. "The average woman needs about twenty minutes of very direct, steady, gentle stimulation of her clitoris to have an orgasm."

I'm not sure where I came up with the *twenty minutes,* but it's my standard recitation. "Some more, some less. And it needs to be steady, not this way and that, changing every few minutes." I figure this covers everyone, and if a woman really gets twenty minutes, she's lucky. If she has an orgasm in ten, she'll just think she's highly sexed.

"Unfortunately," I continue, "the way God or Nature designed the female body, it's hard to get that much stimulation from actual intercourse, even if the guy goes on all night." I use my fingers, like Dr. Ruth does, to demonstrate. "In fact, if he goes on *too* long, you start to get dry and then you *will* hurt."

I pause to let Rebba absorb what I'm saying. "So probably, if you continue on with the oral stimulation or if you use some kind of lubrication and show him what to do with his hands, you'll get more and more excited and eventually come. That's what your body was meant to do. You're young and you're healthy, and you're already excited. I really think it will work."

"I don't know—" The girl starts to argue but stops when I peer over the top of my reading glasses. Rebba screws up her face.

"Really, this is what you have to do," I continue. "If you aren't comfortable asking—what's his name?"

"Andy."

"If you aren't comfortable asking Andy to do it, *show* him with your hand what you like, what feels good. And make a moaning sound when he gets it right. Let him know. I guarantee it will drive him wild."

Rebba shakes her head.

"What?" I ask.

"I couldn't. I . . . I would be too embarrassed."

"Well, then, you will have to practice by yourself."

I purposely don't use the word *masturbate*. So many women have learned it's wrong, but I figure if God gave you something that feels that good, you were meant to use it. Before Rebba has a chance to further object, I leave the exam room and return with a small bag of K-Y samples.

Rebba is standing next to the door, dressed in jeans and a light blue tank top. She is tall and slim with good posture, a willow in spring. "I want you to try what I told you," I say, "five times in the next two weeks, for at least twenty minutes each time. That's just about two hours of your life, and it's for a good cause. I guarantee if you do, eventually you and Andy will be very happy."

I close the exam room door and head down the hall to my office. Sometimes I wonder where I get the balls to talk to women like that, as if I'm some kind of expert.

Sometimes I crack myself up.

Communion

When I'm horny, my legs are restless and I tighten my butt. I never noticed, but Tom teases me about it. We've been buddies so long, we know all each other's moves, know all the moles on each other's backs, and know before the tears come what will make each other cry.

It's my own fault I get horny. I never think about having sex until after eleven, after I've played the piano, done laundry, e-mailed the boys, as I do every few days, and then lain with my husband watching a video or reading aloud. We kiss or mess around a little, but by then I'm so tired, all I want to do is sleep. A few hours later, I'm awake again, staring at the alarm clock, stretching my legs and tightening my butt.

I lie in bed now wondering if Rebba will practice what I told her. I smile in the dark and slide closer to my husband, trying not to wake him, moving my hand between my legs . . . just testing, smelling his sweet man smell. He's so tired tonight. One of his post-op patients dropped her blood pressure, and he came home from the hospital late. He thinks that the woman is stable, but I anticipate the pager will go off through the night. I squirm closer.

Tom isn't asleep. He rolls over to hold me. When I come, I draw him on me with a desperation I've gotten used to but still don't understand.

Then we ride away together past the moon and back into dreams.

SHIANA

Before I open the door, I know the woman is young, a college student, not from Torrington, and scared. I get all this from the first line on the progress note, next to her vital signs.

The name, Shiana Rogers, possibly African American. The insurance, Pennsylvania Alliance, likely out of Philly. The age, nineteen, means she's probably a student, since Torrington, West Virginia, is a college town. The presenting problem, written in Abby's loosely legible scrawl, is *Wants to discuss birth control, and other issues. Patient's first gyn exam.* First exam is how I know the patient is scared. At the first exam they're always scared.

I tap on the door. *Dum-de-dum-dum.* It's my usual friendly knock. Carrying the yellow chart under my arm, I greet the young woman who sits on the gray guest chair in the thin blue exam gown. Her brown arms are folded and her bare legs hang down, not reaching the floor. She has on red socks. "Hi, Shiana, I'm Patsy Harman, nurse-midwife and gyn practitioner. How are you?"

"Good, I guess," she responds in a small voice. I reach out my hand, and the girl takes it, hesitantly, with the tips of her cold fingers. She pulls back, but I hold on. Just for a second.

"This room's a little cold. Your fingers are like ice." The room is not really cold. The patient's just nervous.

I lower myself onto the rolling gray vinyl stool that swivels like the ones at an old-fashioned soda fountain, then I stand, reach into the drawer at the side of the exam table, and pull out a clean white sheet. I wrap it around Shiana's narrow shoulders then settle back down.

Shiana is small, about five foot three, and a little plump. She has smooth coffee-colored skin, dark almond eyes, and straightened black hair pulled away from her face in a ponytail. She's kept her pink baseball cap on. Embroidered with Greek letters, it looks strange with the blue cotton exam gown, but I don't smile. "So, what brings you here today? Is this just an annual checkup or are you having a problem?"

The tears come before the words. I reach for the box of tissues on the counter and scoot the stool closer. I don't speculate, just wait. It could be anything. I've heard so many tearful stories. It doesn't pay to guess.

She surprises me though. "I'm just so *mad!* I'm so mad and embarrassed. I really don't want to be here. I don't want to be anywhere." Shiana catches my eye, then looks away.

I take a deep breath. "It must be pretty bad, but you know what, I've heard a lot of stories in the exam room and—"

"He pulled out and he left it in."

It takes me a minute to figure it out. Pulled out . . . left it in? "A condom?"

"Yes." Very quietly. "We were lying in bed, see, just talking, in the candlelight. It was our first time. I live in the dorm, but my roommate was gone. When I moved to get more comfortable, he rolled over and went to the bathroom. I didn't think that was so strange that he went to the bathroom. I could hear him peeing, but when he came out with his clothes on I asked him, 'Where are you going? Is there something wrong?' and he said, 'I just have to go now.'"

Shiana is talking more to herself than to me. "He didn't kiss me good-bye or anything, he just grabbed his cap off the dresser and left. I felt bad, but I thought, *Well, what a jerk!*" Her almond eyes flash. "But now I know why. He left the condom in me." She looks down. "I tried to get it out, but it's still in there."

I move the stool a little closer. Her voice is so soft, I can hardly hear. "Can you tell me when this happened?"

"Friday night." Shiana looks up at me, tears welling in her eyes. It's now eleven in the morning on Tuesday, much too late for the emergency birth control pill.

"It's okay, Shiana. Come on now; let's start by getting this thing out. Put your feet in these *gadgets.*" I never call them *stirrups.* I have a thing about that. It reminds me of cowboys and cowboy boots with silver spurs. I take the young woman's red-socked feet and guide them into the cloth-covered footrests. "Just slide your bottom down to the end and try not to be embarrassed. I can get the condom out, and then you'll feel better and we'll talk about what else we should do."

It isn't very difficult. The condom is wadded behind the cervix. I find it with a gloved index finger and work it toward the opening. Then I grab it with a ring forceps. It smells about like you'd think a four-day-old condom with semen in it would smell, and it's bright blue.

I don't say anything about the odor. The girl knows. I bury it deep in the trash and secure the stainless-steel lid. "If you don't mind, Shiana, I think I should check you for infection, since you're here. I know this is your first exam so I'll be real careful. It won't hurt."

"Go ahead," says the girl, "I want to be checked for everything. I was always so careful . . . I never did it without a condom. *Ever.* I know some girls do."

I put the swab in a tube so I can send it to the lab and have them test for gonorrhea and chlamydia. There are other tests that need to be done. Some results don't come back for days. Some infections take weeks or years to appear. Some have no treatment. Some are deadly. The girl knows this. She's always used condoms.

While I work I ask Shiana where she's from. It's my habit to keep the women talking so they won't be so nervous. She isn't from Philly. She's from Erie. Her mom's a teacher. Her dad's in business. They don't know she's sexually active. "They would die."

Shiana wipes her face with her hands. She has a silver ring on every finger. She lies squinting at the ceiling while tears run down the sides of her soft brown cheeks. I want to take her in my arms and hold her, but I'm afraid my warmth would scare her away.

When I'm finished, I fill out the lab slip. We'll get tests for everything: gonorrhea, chlamydia, hepatitis, syphilis, herpes, and HIV. In a few weeks, some may need to be repeated. It's too early for a pregnancy check. That's a wait-and-pray item.

Shiana's period is due in two weeks. Very bad timing. If she has a regular twenty-eight-day cycle, she may already have ovulated. Still, the young woman might get lucky. I'm not sure how a wadded-up condom will affect sperm motility, probably slow them down some.

When the lab slip is filled out, I seat myself again on the round swivel stool. "This was a hard thing that happened," I say. "Some guys are assholes.

"The nurse will call you with the results of the tests. It will take a few days. I'll give you antibiotics as a precaution, but they won't treat every infection. They won't cover a virus. Do you think you should start birth control pills? You know, just as a precaution for next time?"

"There won't be a *next time*," Shiana mutters, then lights the room up with a grin. It's her first smile, and I see the outgoing, optimistic person she used to be, the woman before the condom. "Or at least not for a *long time*," she continues. "I'm through with men."

I smile. "Well, if you don't get your period in three weeks, come back and see me. We'll do a pregnancy test and I'll help you figure out what to do." Shiana has no one to tell. No one else to talk to. Not her mother: "No way!" Or sorority sisters: "It's so humiliating . . ." So the *we* means a lot.

I walk Shiana to the checkout desk with my arm around her like we're old friends.

Plague of Locusts

The thought of the twenty-one-thousand-dollar IRS debt rests like a stone in the bottom of my stomach, and I sit on the porch with my jam jar of booze, wondering if I've tried hard enough to go back to sleep. In the moonlight I can just see the shadow of the gazebo with the purple clematis climbing the rail. I can't see the asparagus pushing up in the garden. I can't see the peach tree now in full bloom.

It's not just the money. It's our being inept. We should have known, should have kept better track. But we're always so busy, so tired. And then, let's face it, if it comes to rechecking an accountant's figures or sitting on the porch and watching an osprey soar in circles over Hope Lake, you know what we choose. In my worst frame of mind I call us airhead hippies. I said this to Tom and it pissed him off.

I'm tired of trying so hard, but it's not like we have a choice now. We can't walk away. If the practice doesn't survive, Tom and I will still be responsible for the twenty-one thousand dollars we may owe the IRS, as well as all the money we borrowed: the fifty thousand dollars to start up the practice, the forty thousand dollars for the laser equipment, the sixty-five thousand dollars for the ultrasound machine, and the seventy thousand dollars to purchase the mandatory OB insurance policy tail, which will cover us for the next eighteen years for any prior acts of alleged obstetrical negligence.

I feel like I'm always running in front of a plague of locusts, running to see patients, running to promote the practice, running to keep ahead of the bills. This past year, Tom has worked longer and longer hours, asking the secretaries to keep his surgical schedule full. Each day we get home later. The cost of salaries, employee benefits, and rent for the office goes up, while what insurance companies pay keeps plummeting.

Rebecca Gorham e-mailed today that she found someone in the Cleveland IRS office who's willing to review our case. She'll meet with him at the end of the week. I'm hoping they'll find it's an error. If they don't, I've no clue what we'll do.

"What the hell." I take a sip of the sleep medicine. When a breeze wakens the wind chimes, I can smell   peach blossoms, and my stomach relaxes around the warm scotch.

This night of blossoms is my world, not the worry and hassle of running a practice. I rise heavily and lean over the rail. Rain was predicted, but the moon floats in and out of the clouds.

Saluting all that is good and uncomplicated, I raise my hands to the sky.

CHAPTER 3

Forever and Ever, Amen

"Did you see that girl?" Linda asks. "The one with the purple hair?"

"Which one?" I kid her, like there were three. She gives me a look. The secretary's frizzy red hair bounces when she talks. I'm at the microwave in the clinic kitchen, heating up lentils.

"The young woman with the two kids. The hippie chick."

"You couldn't help noticing." Donna pops open her soda. "Not just the hair, but she sat right there in the waiting room with her boob hanging out." Everyone snickers.

"Her breast? Why?"

"She was feeding the kid," chimes in Linda.

"Well there's nothing wrong with her breast-feeding here," I respond. "This is a women's health practice."

Donna rolls her eyes. "But the kid must have been three years old. He could practically read!"

I'm settling down with the staff for lunch. I usually eat in my office next to a stack of unfinished charts, but I've caught up with my work for a change. I can take a few minutes to relax. The kitchen is small. There's room only for a white table, a fridge, and a sink. Today everyone has gone out to eat except Linda, Donna, and our junior receptionist, Junie. They've brought their cafeteria trays back from the hospital and are opening drinks, reaching for napkins and condiments.

I dip into my homemade bean soup, surreptitiously checking out my officemates' selections. The array of fried food amazes me: fried chicken fingers, fried cheese, and french fries. For dessert, there's chocolate cake. It's not that it doesn't smell good, but where are the veggies? I don't say anything, just munch on my baby carrots.

"So, you were a hippie, weren't you?" asks Linda, stretching across for the salt. She's been with the practice almost since it began, and loves to get me going. "Did you have purple hair?"

I wink at Junie, the new staff member, twenty-one and a little bit of a hippie herself, a kindred spirit. "I'm still a hippie, at heart, anyway." Today all three of the women wear lavender gingham scrubs, but Junie has a huge rhinestone brooch pinned to hers. The girl has flair, I'll give her that.

"Tell Junie how you and Dr. Harman got married," Linda persists. "You were naked in a field of daisies, right?"

I shake my head. The three look at me, expecting a story, and I feel like an elder sitting down at a campfire.

"It *was* in a field of daisies," I begin. "We lived on the commune then. You've heard about this, Junie?" The youngest woman nods. "It was down near Spencer. We lived on top of a beautiful ridge with a group of other peaceniks. Tom had asked me probably twenty times if I'd marry him. I'd always said no. My parents were divorced, and I figured if we got married we'd just break up like everyone else. If we stayed lovers, there might be a chance." Donna nods, understanding.

"You said no?" Linda's heard this before.

"Yeah, I said no all those times, then this one day . . . We slept in a tent with a wooden floor. We called it the butterfly tent because it was in a field of daisies and butterfly weeds. You know that flower, the butterfly weed? It's bright orange and blooms in midsummer.

"Well, this day, Dr. Harman was sick, running a high fever, with chills. We didn't have a thermometer then. He was probably about one hundred and three, but he wasn't a doctor, remember, just a scrawny hippie with a beard and long hair. I wasn't a nurse or a midwife. I think it might have been a kidney infection, but we didn't have health insurance, so we made herbal teas, drank lots of fluids, waited it out.

"So, this one day he looks up at me when he's all pale and sweaty and he says, 'Will you marry me?' This must have been the twenty-first time . . . I wasn't counting. He looked pitiful, really. I'm sitting in the hot tent in June wringing out warm compresses for his back and for some reason I smile and say, 'Yeah.' That's all, just 'Yeah.'

"The next morning we wake up. The fever had broken, and he felt weak but lots better. We were lying in the tent looking out the netting at daisies and orange butterfly flowers and monarchs flitting around, and I asked him, 'So, are we married?'

"And he said, 'Yep.'

"And I said, looking into his eyes, 'Forever?' and he said, 'Yep.'

"And that was it. A few months later we went to a friend who was a priest and he made it legal, but in our hearts it happened that day. Later I realized it was Friday the thirteenth, but we've been together now for almost thirty years, so I guess it was lucky for us." I stand up, signaling the story has come to an end.

Everyone sighs. "So were you naked?" Donna asks with a twinkle, coiling her long brown hair up in a French twist.

"Yes," I say as I bag up my soup container and wipe off my place at the table, "I imagine we were."

KASMAR

"Hi, Kasmar. Am I saying that right? How are you today?" The freckle-faced woman nods and flashes a tight smile. She's dressed in the blue exam gown and her clothes are piled neatly on the guest chair. I reach out my hand before I sit down and she takes it firmly.

Reading the history clipped to the front of Kasmar Layton's chart, you wouldn't know there was anything remarkable about her. She's forty-eight, already through menopause, apparently healthy; no bowel, bladder, or sexual problems; never smoked, eats a low-fat diet, and teaches horticulture at Torrington University's School of Agriculture. She's a new patient and here for her annual exam.

I'm on a roll today, hoping to be out of the office early. I need to pack tonight, and I have to go to the bank, the pharmacy, and the supermarket for dog food. Tomorrow Tom and I and Roscoe, our short basset-beagle, will leave for a long weekend at our Lake Erie cottage.

I palpate the patient's breasts. "So when did you have the breast reduction? Recently?" Wide white scars make crosses below the nipples on both sides.

"Two years ago."

"Were you happy you did it?"

"Yes. It's something I always wanted to do and I finally got up my nerve. I wish I'd had them made smaller though. I hate to think of going back for another surgery." I'm mildly surprised. Her breasts are already cup size A.

"Do you do your own breast exam?"

"Yes."

I assist Kasmar to place her feet in the covered footrests, then put on my gloves and sit between her legs, adjusting the exam sheet so I can still see her face. "You can pull down the pillow if you want." The woman appears tense but reaches above her head with both hands and adjusts the flowered pillow, smoothing her close-cropped black curls. Kasmar wears no makeup and no jewelry. She's pretty in an angular way: high cheekbones, arched eyebrows over blue eyes, a long face with a prominent jaw; a good strong face.

First I inspect the outside of the patient's genitals. The labia are small and dry, a sign of decreased estrogen. "Are you married, Kasmar?"

"I have a long-term partner."

The vagina's so tiny I use the smallest speculum, watching the patient's face as I carefully open it. "Do you have intercourse regularly?"

"Not very often." Kasmar grimaces. You can tell the exam hurts, but she doesn't move or make noise. She's one tough lady. I appreciate this.

"You doing okay?"

"Yeah." Kasmar stares at the ceiling.

Finished with the exam, I assist the patient to a sitting position and hand her the box of tissues. "Well, everything seems fine. You did great. Your vagina's a little dry and tight, though. Does it hurt when you make love?"

"No."

"Are you sure? Because there's an estrogen cream I could prescribe. It's very effective with problems like this."

"It's not a problem." The patient flinches and pinches her mouth shut.

I drop the subject. The woman and her husband must have come to some agreement about sex. "Why don't you get dressed and I'll fill out your mammogram requisition." I slip out the door and check my watch, smiling. Fifteen minutes from start to finish. If I could do this more often I might get to leave on time in the evening, like the other nurse-practitioners.

When I return to the exam room, Kasmar is waiting, dressed in a soft blue long-sleeved shirt and navy slacks with black heavy-soled walking shoes. It's the kind of outfit you might expect a horticulture professor to wear; she looks ready to go out into the fields to inspect the tassels of corn. Opening her leather briefcase, Kasmar removes a file. "I want to discuss a few things with you, if you don't mind."

Shit, I was doing so well. I return to my stool. This could be anything.

"I wanted to get that over so that I could talk to you." She takes a big breath. "I really hate those exams. They make me so tense. But I need to get this out in the air . . . I'm a lesbian. My partner is a woman. I think you know her, Jerry Slater?"

I do a double take like in the cartoons but keep my face impassive. I hope it's impassive. First I recall Jerry Slater, a petite graying blond who teaches nursing at the university. Surely not! I can't remember the details of her face, but I recall a gentle, sweet woman. I contemplate Kasmar in a new way. "I do remember her. She's been in a few times. Is she the person who referred you?"

"Yeah, she and my therapist, Karen Rossi. You know her?" I nod. Karen is a woman in my meditation group. "I needed a checkup, but I also wanted to present something to you. I've been attending the Persad Center for Diversity in Pittsburgh for the last three years." She announces this as if it's significant and I should know what that means.

"Persid? Persidio?" It doesn't ring a bell, but then I don't get up to the city that often. It must be some kind of support group. "I'm afraid I'm not familiar with that organization."

"It's the Center for Transgender Therapy."

I'm still slow getting the drift.

Kasmar continues, "I want to become a man and I was hoping you could assist me."

I can't help it, my eyes widen.

"I've been going to counseling for a long time and I feel it's what I was meant to be. These are letters of support from my therapist and my doctors in Pittsburgh." She hands over the two manila files. "What I need is someone locally who can prescribe the testosterone and do the follow-up exams and labs for me." She waits for my response.

"You know, this is something that's never come up before," I say, stalling. I'm thinking women do all sorts of things to themselves. They get nose jobs, boob jobs, and dye their hair blue. They pierce their nipples. They have cellulite removed and lips plumped up. We do laser treatments for the removal of unwanted hair and spider veins in our office. Is this so different?

"My husband's a surgeon, but I d-don't think he's qualified . . ." I stutter. "I've never been asked this before."

"I'm not surprised." Kasmar responds with her first real smile. She has a wide generous mouth, soft lips, and white teeth. "I'm not planning on surgery at this point."

I clear my throat. "And you're *sure* you want to do this? There are potential risks to high doses of testosterone. You know that?"

"I do. But I also have a complete protocol from the Gender Dysphoria Association." She hands over a thick document entitled "Standard of Care for Gender Identity Disorders, Sixth Version." I glance at the cover. Committee authors include ten MDs, six PhDs, a physician's assistant, and a doctor of public health. The index indicates that the manuscript has chapters on the initial labs, the exam schedule, the follow-up labs, and the graduated doses of testosterone injections.

I hate to ask again, but I do. "And you're *sure* you want to do this?"

She doesn't hesitate. "I *am* going to do this. Once I made the decision I felt a huge weight lift off me, a feeling of hope that I could be free of a mask I've always worn. I wasn't meant to be a woman. I'm sure of it. It just took me nearly forty years to come to that conclusion."

"And you've talked to your partner?"

"Jerry's gone to some of my therapy sessions and is supportive."

"What about your family, do your parents understand? I know you're a grown woman and they can't stop you, but do they understand?"

"My mom's dead. She died a few years ago. My dad understands."

"And why again do you want *us* to help you? Couldn't you go to Pittsburgh?"

"I will if you say no, but it's a three-hour drive and then another forty-five minutes across the city. I figured I would have to take a day off work for each visit, and at first I'm supposed to come once a month. I thought I would ask you because Jerry said you were open-minded . . . I just thought I would ask." There are no tears. She's not begging. It took a lot of courage for her to disclose her plan.

I could say no and be done with it, as I imagine most providers in Torrington would, but I hedge instead. I need to think this over carefully. "You know, this is something I want to consult with Dr. Harman about. I'll ask him to read over the protocols and see what he thinks. I'll tell him you seem like a thoughtful and intelligent woman."

"Tell him I'm Jerry's husband. He knows her. He did a laparoscopy on her a few years ago for an ovarian cyst. I met him at the hospital." *Jerry's husband,* I mentally echo.

Standing, I reach for Kasmar's hand and shake it. "It's not that I have any judgment against this, you understand. I just have to sort it all out. Can I get back to you in a few weeks? I want to do some research and I want to talk to Dr. Harman."

"That's fine."

I watch the patient walk down the long white hall as she leaves. Is it true what I said, that I don't have any judgment against it?

Kasmar is tall and thin, with narrow hips and a long stride. From the back she *could* be a man. Inside she already is.

Searchlight

I don't write down the patients' stories every night, the stories they tell in the exam room. Some nights I sleep. Not many. Some nights I write poetry in a worn spiral notebook. Some nights I go over the practice's low bank account or lie on my back in the dark and worry about our three mostly grown boys. My mind works like a searchlight, moving back and forth through the shadows, looking for trouble.

Tonight I wander the living room in my white robe like a ghost, worrying about Orion. This is my middle son's first year in the master of fine arts program at the University of Cincinnati. His live-in girlfriend of seven years, Lucy, left him six months ago. He's alone in a place where he knows hardly anyone, and he's still mourning her loss.

Zen, at the College of Santa Fe, asks for spending money too often but is doing okay. Tom's been tight with the handouts, told him to get a part-time job, but that's hard when he's taking so many credits.

I turn my beam on Mica. He's settled in Atlanta with his fiancée, Emma, and he's unemployed but never asks for help. I'm not sure what he lives on. He does some Internet consulting occasionally but hasn't phoned or e-mailed for weeks.

I hate telephoning my oldest son. When I get his answering machine, I'm afraid I'll sound like a mother in a sitcom. "Hi, Mica," the recording will say in a thin nasal whine. "It's your *mom* calling, for the sixth time." I can picture him deleting my messages and rolling his eyes. I take a deep breath. He would call if he needed me, wouldn't he?

There was a dark time for us when Mica was fourteen. Tom and I had left the farm to go back to school, and for two years our oldest went back and forth between the commune on the ridge and our home in Ohio. When we moved to Minnesota so I could go to the graduate program in midwifery, he refused to come. He wanted to stay in West Virginia with his biological father, Stacy. It made sense in a way. He'd grown up there. All his friends were in Spencer. Why would he want to be dragged around the country and attend school in a different place each year? But I missed him so.

That's when I started the long conversations on my knees with God. "Protect my boys. Shine your light on them." For almost two years we had no contact with Mica. I would write a letter every week, but he never answered, and I never knew if he got them. There was no phone on what was left of the commune. It was as if the child I had breast-fed for twenty-four months, read countless stories to, taught how to tie his shoes, was dead. Then, almost as suddenly as he left us, he rose from the grave. We started seeing him on weekends when Tom began medical school at Ohio State in Columbus.

Now whenever I don't hear from Mica for a month, I fear he will disappear again forever. Like tonight. I pace the porch missing him and worrying about him . . .

I'm making myself sick thinking like this! I gulp down the scotch and go back to the bedroom. As I pass the dresser, I feel in the dark for the small red prayer box and place my hand on the round wooden lid.

TRISH

"Do you have a minute?"

I look up at the clock. It's one thirty in the afternoon, and I'm just finishing charts in my office. If Tom and I don't leave by three, we'll miss the ferry to the island, but Trish is my friend, and even if she weren't, I'd pull up the guest chair and close the door with my foot, as I do now. "What's up?"

Trish sits but doesn't say anything. Then quietly, "Aran's pregnant." There are tears in her eyes. "She's been sexually active since she was sixteen, but she's always taken birth control pills. It's exactly what happened to me. I was planning to go to college and took my pills every day. I got pregnant at seventeen too." Trish wipes her lightly freckled face with the back of her hand. "I guess we're just fertile." A weak smile. "It's Jimmy. He's the father. The one she went to the prom with. You know how Dan feels. He thinks the kid's bad news, into drugs. I think he's okay, maybe a little lazy, maybe just immature." Trish never says anything bad about anyone, so her characterizing Jimmy as lazy is saying a lot. My friend's straight sandy hair is parted to the side; she's a sweet-looking woman with a soft oval face. She stares over my head out the window, then continues.

"Aran's a little on the wild side but she's an A student. She's already been accepted at State with a full scholarship." Trish pauses and runs her hands over her flowered scrub top, smoothing the wrinkles. I notice her name tag is crooked. "I make an effort to like Jimmy, I really do."

She clears her throat. "I've been trying to go easy on Aran. She feels so bad. She said she was never going to have kids, and now this. And she's not just a *little* pregnant. She's been hiding it. I bet she's four months along. She was afraid to tell us, just wore baggy clothes, and I didn't notice. Dan found out last night when one of her friends made a comment." Trish laughs bitterly. "I think what hurts most is she didn't tell us."

I study my friend as she gazes out the window at a sky filled with rolling gray clouds. She rocks back and forth as if cradling a baby. There isn't a sound in the office.

Aran's probably already in her second trimester, past the point of miscarrying or considering a termination. She won't be going to college next year. Maybe any year. She'll lose her scholarship. Trish and Dan live month to month. They've been fixing up a three-bedroom ranch house on Perry Mountain. They have an eight year old, an eleven-year-old, a seventeen-year-old . . . and soon a new baby. There will be no money for the university.

"Do you think they'll get married?" I ask.

"I've been thinking about that. I hope not. I don't want her to rush into it just because of the baby. If it doesn't work out she'll have to get a divorce. Truthfully, we haven't talked about it yet. We haven't talked *at all*. After everything came out, Dan slammed the door and went into the garage. He didn't come to bed until midnight, and Aran locked herself in her room. He left for work early and then Aran got on the school bus."

"Have you told anyone else yet?"

"No. I couldn't. I couldn't without crying. I wanted to tell you first, so I waited until the office was closed and you'd be alone. I just feel so sad. Aran wanted so bad to go to college. She would have been the first in my family."

I take a long breath. "So will Aran come see me?"

"She's still on my insurance, but I don't think it covers obstetrics."

"It doesn't matter about insurance. You know it doesn't. I'll get her an appointment when I get back from Canada. Did I tell you we're going to the island? If my schedule is full, I'll see her at five on Tuesday." We stand up, holding on to each other. Trish's head comes just up to my shoulder.

If I had known then the pain that was coming, maybe I would have done something different. But you never know, do you? You can't see it coming. The seeds of love and despair were already planted, already sown, like an embryo growing, or maybe a cancer.

Earth Dream

Somewhere between Cleveland and Sandusky, along the tollway where it stretches flat against the heartland, I start to nod off. Tom expects this and finds an oldies rock-and-roll station coming out of Oberlin. I pat him on the leg. "Just gonna take a little nap . . ." He smiles, knowing how I am. I don't sleep well in bed at night, but put me in a warm car in the passenger seat and I sleep like a baby. I wake when we get to the ferry dock, trying to hold on to the dream:

An old woman wearing a long white dress sits at the side of a garden. In her basket are children, miniature children, toddlers to teens. My boys are there too, little blond boys, now really men. I sit down beside her.

What have you learned? I ask the wise crone.

Her voice is the sound of water flowing over stone.

The sun rises. The sun sets. We do not need to hold it up.

The river flows downhill. We can swim with it or against. Spring always comes.

The river flows downhill and I am swimming against it.

*

Summer

CHAPTER 4

Liberation

A low rumble as the ferry plows through dark waves, and the smell of diesel exhaust. I love this two-hour ride across Lake Erie. Usually we come in the daylight when we can see the other islands: Kelleys, South Bass, and Middle Bass Island. Tonight we see only the lights of cottages on the black masses that jut up from the lower basin of the huge freshwater inland sea. There's something beautiful and exotic about the darkness and the water. We could be off the coast of France, but we're only five hours from Torrington.

I take a deep breath and let it out slowly, let the weight of the past few months blow into the wind. Officially it's not summer yet, but our first trip of the year to the Pelee is always summer for me. I'm looking forward to the long weekend at our cottage, which sits on the southern shore of Pelee Island, the southernmost tip of Canada.

"You cold?" Tom asks, putting his arm around my waist and pulling me over. "I could go down to the car and get you a sweater."

"No, I'm fine." I snuggle up to him. I always feel like we're coming home when we go to the island. Something unwinds inside me.

An hour later, at the front door of the big yellow farmhouse, we scratch around in the flower bed, searching for the key. There are no street lamps, no ambient lighting, just the wide stretch of lawn and the trees and the starlight. I always forget which rock the key's under. Tom always remembers. Just inside the door he finds the switch and flicks on the overhead. Blinking into the white, I see the familiar photographs arranged on the shelves along the family room wall, years of vacations captured in mismatched frames. Images of our three boys fishing, boys eating at picnic tables, boys on the ferry boat, boys playing in the water, boys dunking their father. There's even a few of my husband and me.

Tom drags in our bag and a small red cooler. The beds are already made with the colorful quilts I collect. Canned food is stored in the pine cupboards. All we have to do is put the milk in the fridge and open a bottle of wine.

I check out the house while Tom digs around in the drawer for the corkscrew. The kitchen is tidy. The big table that seats ten has the same vinyl lace tablecloth that I put on last fall. The housekeepers are doing a good job, and the weekly summer renters are being kind to the place. I pull the blinds up and continue my inspection. Even though it's dark tonight, I want to see the sun and the lake in the morning.

In the living room, the sofa and love seat are covered with matching green quilts. My photographs cover the walls, and Tom's pottery is displayed on the built-in shelves. I open the sliding glass door to let in some air and open the windows in the big downstairs bedroom where my favorite blue patchwork is spread over the bed.

"You ready?" Tom yells.

"Coming."

As we climb up the steps to the deck on the break wall I almost trip. One board is loose, and Tom says he'll fix it in the morning. He carries the wine. I can smell that our two acres of grass have been mown by our local handyman just today.

In front of us is water, twenty miles of water, and far in the distance are the lights from small towns on the U.S. side. Tom grew up in northwest Ohio. He can point out Port Clinton, Marblehead, and Vermilion. With his parents and two brothers, he lived in the house in Fostoria on Colonial Drive until he was eighteen. The same house. The same bed. Even now, when we visit, nothing has changed. The silverware and waxed paper are in the exact same drawers.

Tom's father was a welder at the Union Carbide factory. His mother was a stay-at-home mom who volunteered for the Red Cross and led a Boy Scout troop. The family fished these waters, pulling up thousands of perch, walleye, and bass. I think sometimes that it's Tom's secure upbringing that gives him his optimism, the same way my background makes me wait for something to go wrong.

We sit quietly on the deck, taking in the smell of fish and grass, no car noises, no voices, just crickets and water and wind. We watch the sky, watch the sliver of moon and the clouds as they open and close around it.

I break the silence. "Had an interesting patient this morning."

Tom groans. "Can't you ever stop thinking about work, Patsy? Give it up."

"No, really, this is interesting."

"Okay," he says with a grunt, filling our wineglasses a second time and scooting his chair closer to the railing

"She wants to become a man. She wants us to help her."

Tom chuckles. I see the flash of his teeth when he smiles into the dark. "What did you say?"

"That I'd think about it and talk to you."

"I don't do that kind of surgery. She'd be better off in Cleveland. I know someone who does it. Remember? When I was a resident there I assisted Dr. Ernest with making a vagina into a penis."

"My patient doesn't want surgery. She just needs help with the testosterone injections and labs. It's all organized through some center in Pittsburgh. She gave me a protocol that tells what labs to draw to be sure there aren't any serious side effects and gives all the technical information about the injections."

"Why doesn't she just go to Pittsburgh then? Why'd she come to us?"

"Her significant other is our patient. You remember a woman named Jerry Slater? I think that was it . . . Kasmar says she met you at the hospital when you did Jerry's surgery. She says she's Jerry's *husband*. Does that ring a bell?"

"Sure, I did a scope on Jerry for a cyst last year. She's a nurse at the university hospital. That tall, thin woman's her partner? I didn't even know Jerry was gay." Tom remembers everyone's name. Phone numbers, even.

"Come on! You can't tell by looking. I could be gay," I tease him.

"Right," Tom says and laughs, trying to pinch my nipple through my sweatshirt. He's on target.

"Okay, now, listen. What do you think? Should we do it?" I hold him back with one hand.

"You're serious? Why would we?"

"Because she's a nice person, and if we help her she won't have to drive all the way to Pittsburgh each month."

"You like her? How old is she?" Tom rises to peer down into the churning water.

"Yeah, I do. She seems intelligent and committed . . . about forty-seven, I think. I admire her. My only concern is metaphysical. Is it right? Is it messing too much with nature?"

"People do a lot weirder things. Will she be hurting anyone?" He turns to me.

I shake my head no.

"Well then, it's a free country. I think we should help her. Who else in Torrington will?" Tom slides his gaze back to the distant shore and lifts his wineglass up to the sky. Fireworks are going off in the distance at Cedar Point Amusement Park, as they do at ten every night in the summer. The waves crash below us under the deck.

I lean against him and lift my glass too.

ARAN

On Tuesday morning, back home, sitting on the porch holding my morning coffee, I sight the first Baltimore oriole of the season, a blaze of fire on the top of the peach tree. An hour later, in the clinic, I scan my schedule for Trish's daughter's name and find it in an improvised slot at the end of the day.

At five, I knock on the exam room door, a new chart for Aran under my arm. I see a petite young woman with the same sandy blond hair as her mother, but cut very short. She has an unblemished face and three silver studs in each ear. The boyfriend, a solemn, stocky eighteen-year-old with buzz-cut red hair and thick eyebrows, slouches low in the guest chair. As I step by, he moves his black army boots out of the way.

I go through the usual introductions and then get down to business. "Aran, I know this pregnancy isn't what you expected. Your mom told me you'd never planned to have children. It must be a hard adjustment. You doing okay?"

"I guess . . ." Aran doesn't look up. Her pink flip-flops hang from her toes.

"Do you think you're going to be able to handle it? Because there are alternatives. If you aren't already too far along you could have a termination or think about giving the baby up for adoption. You're pretty young to be a mom."

"I could never do that!" Aran says adamantly, now looking straight at me. Her blue eyes flash. "I don't believe in abortion unless there's something wrong with the baby, and I wouldn't consider adoption. How would I know if the baby got a good home or was being abused?"

"You could contact an adoption agency. All the prospective parents are carefully screened." Jimmy is shaking his head no, but he still hasn't spoken.

I decide I've gone on enough about alternatives. Clearly, they won't consider them, and I don't want to push it. After the physical exam and the review of the information in the OB packet, I take the couple down the hall to the ultrasound room for an unofficial scan. As I'm typing in Aran's demographics, there's a tap at the door. "Can I watch too?" Trish pokes her head into the darkened room. Abby, my nurse, must have called her to come up from the family medicine suite just in time.

"Okay with you?" I ask her daughter. The girl shrugs. The three of them, Aran, Jimmy, and Trish, stare at the screen as unidentifiable shapes swirl around and I get my bearings. I'm not a whiz at ultrasound but I can usually find the embryo's heartbeat. "There's the fetus." I point to the flicker of white life. "See its heart beating?" Aran and Jimmy stare at the screen without expression. Maybe they were hoping this whole thing was a mistake, that there wasn't really a baby, that it was just going to go away.

Trish tries hard to be upbeat. With appropriate enthusiasm she says, "Well, hi there, little fellow." The fetus raises its arm and waves. "He *is* an active one!" Then the room is dead silent. Nobody else says *anything*.

When I glance up from the monitor to turn on the lights, I'm surprised to see Jimmy wiping his eyes.

Courage

It's 2:00 a.m. and I'm still not asleep. I turn on my side, inspecting the stained-glass mandala that hangs in the window at the peak of the high ceiling, then I plump another pillow under my head. The full moon moves in and out of the clouds. This bedroom is a big box of moonlight. It's so large, our whole log cabin at the farm would fit in the space. All over the world, families of ten live in houses smaller than this room.

I'm worried about Aran. I wish she would look into adoption. In this part of Appalachia, neither abortion nor adoption is seriously considered. There's a strong feeling for family. Kin will take care of kin.

Though it's rare for a mother in West Virginia to give up her baby, I've always thought it one of the noblest things a woman can do. And one of the hardest. I pad out to the porch with my dose of scotch and sit looking across the lawn toward the gazebo. Two deer stand under the peach tree. I recall one young mother . . .

She was twenty, unmarried, a college student. What was her name, Kari or Karen? She and her boyfriend came for every prenatal visit, and just like any other couple they got excited to hear the heartbeat, excited to see the baby on the ultrasound. By her seventh month she'd already visited a social worker and arranged for a placement.

During the delivery of a baby that's going to be given up, you have to be careful with the words that you use. You don't whisper to the woman in great pain while you hold her, "Think about *your baby*. Your baby will be here soon." You don't urge when she's pushing, "Come on, Mom, you can do it!" And you don't exclaim when you lay the wet infant on her chest, "Congratulations, you're a mother!"

If you say anything at all as you hand the infant to the waiting RN, you quietly declare, "The baby's doing great. It looks healthy." You don't even mention the sex. Then the nurse wheels him or her out in a bassinet, and the room is so quiet you can hear the moaning of the woman still in labor next door.

❊ ❊ ❊

The day of Kari's discharge, after she's had the baby, my patient and her boyfriend ask over the intercom for the infant to be brought to their room. The RNs at the nurses' station look at one another knowingly, thinking the young couple will change their minds and refuse to relinquish. That's what you call it when you give a baby up for adoption, *relinquish*. We've seen young women change their minds at the last minute, more often than not. The baby is brought to the young couple. At two o'clock, the light over their door starts blinking again.

I rise from the desk and drag down the hall, not in a hurry to get there. A couple like this, in college but with family support, could do all right taking a baby home. However, if they do that, an adoptive mother and father who've been expecting to bring home their infant tonight will feel that the baby they've carried near their hearts for months has died.

I knock quietly, and Kari pushes the bassinet to the door. She stands in her green-striped hospital robe with the boyfriend touching her arm. "You can take him now," Kari says, her face red from crying. "We're done saying good-bye." Then she reaches into the bed and pulls the blue flannel blanket up to the tiny boy's neck. The father—he is about the same age as my youngest son—puts a small stuffed monkey in the bassinet. I take both their hands and stand with them for a few minutes saying a prayer, then I roll the cart down the hall . . . It still brings tears to my eyes.

❋   ❋   ❋

The scotch has kicked in and the moon is already sinking into the lake on a stream of silver. I rest my head on the rail. The couple had made the baby by accident and given him away on purpose, a gift to a family that couldn't conceive. At the foot of our bed, I drop my robe to the floor and slide in beside Tom's big, warm body.

I've never forgotten their courage.

Affliction

By dawn I've vomited three times. My husband still sleeps, but I'm pacing the floor. When the pain moves into my chest and I throw up again, I can't put it off any longer. I sit on the side of the bed. "Tom, we have to go to the emergency room."

"What?"

"We have to go to the ER. I've been up since three. It was abdominal pain at first, but now it's up here." I press my fist to my chest. We're both thinking the same thing. *Heart attack.* We dress quickly, say nothing.

If it hadn't been Friday, I would have gone to the ER hours ago. But on Friday night in a college town, it's nothing but drunks and overdoses. When we get there we have to wait anyway. I moan, holding my stomach. "I think I'm going to throw up," I tell Tom. He taps on the window and says three magic words, *chest pain* and *vomit,* and an orderly comes quickly to get me. Then a team in blue scrubs whips into action.

Cold sticky pads are pressed on my chest. An oxygen cannula is placed in my nose, and an overweight male nurse gets the IV in with one try. My stomach is hurting so bad, I don't even notice the pinch of the needle. The doc glances up from the EKG readout. "It's normal," she says to no one. So it's not a heart attack after all. I ask for a sip of water.

I've never had heart trouble before, have never been sick except for the usual colds and seasonal viruses. But this time, I was sure it was *the big one.* Whole grains and veggies are protective up to a point, but stress and guilt have a way of catching up with you.

Soon I'm given some IV Nubain for the pain and I'm floating three feet above my bed. I watch from my perch as a bevy of nurses wanders over to say hello to my husband. The tall blonde, whose name tag says CAROL, swishes her shiny, straight hair and announces that she's made coffee in the doctors' lounge. I can tell Tom's one of their favorites and wonder if it's anything more than that . . . My inner eye squints, watching them chatter.

Tom's short gray hair is receding, but his face is still young. I check him out as a single woman might. Not a bad-looking guy, a straight nose and straight teeth, broad shoulders, nice hands. He could lose a few pounds, but only a wife would notice.

The nurses are laughing at something he's said. Tom's not really flirting. I doubt he knows how. He's just so damn good-humored, all women like him. My eyelids are drooping and . . . and then the medication wears off. The pain is back.

The doctor in a rumpled white lab coat, who is probably the same age as Orion, my middle son, comes by to discharge me. I remember her now. I helped her deliver her first baby, my hands over hers, at the university hospital when she was in med school.

"Your heart's fine and all your labs are normal," she tells us, looking at Tom. "The X-ray shows a hiatal hernia, a weakness in the diaphragm that allows the stomach to expand into the chest." She turns to me. "Did you know that?" Her breath smells of coffee and exhaustion.

"No, not really. I've never had any trouble before. I had bad acid indigestion when I was pregnant years ago." She nods, as if reflux when I was expecting confirms her diagnosis.

It all sounds too simple, but I'm relieved. If I go home and don't eat for a few days, the pain will go away.

I'm not dying after all.

❧   ❧   ❧

The pain does get better, but after three days it hasn't gone away. I still feel the fist in my chest, my temp is 103, and I'm sent back to the hospital for more tests. Everything blurs after that. I'm starting to chill, but getting the CT isn't as bad as I expected. The tech, a man with greased-back hair and braces, says they're going to get a "wet reading" in the next half hour. Tom is in the office seeing patients, and I just want to go home and lie down, so I dress and find my car in the ER parking lot. Twenty minutes later, as I'm crossing the bridge over Hope Lake, my cell phone goes off. I consider ignoring it—I'm sick, for God's sake!—but dutifully pull onto the berm. The phone has stopped ringing but I check the caller ID and return the call.

"Monroe, radiology," a clipped bass voice answers. I picture a dark-eyed, opinionated man I met once at a hospital holiday party.

"Patsy Harman, nurse-midwife, you called?" I respond just as formally.

"Where are you?"

"What . . . ? I'm in my car, almost home."

"Well, you better come back," Monroe growls. "I could be wrong, but I think you have a gangrenous gallbladder."

Gangrene in my gallbladder? I blink, not knowing how to respond. "Okay, where should I go?"

"OR admissions, third floor. You know where that is? I'll call Jamison, the general surgeon. They'll fit you in as an emergency case. He'll meet you there, and I mean now!" This man must have been in the military.

Speed-dialing the office while I'm driving, I take the entrance back onto the freeway too fast, and the rear of the Civic swings out in the gravel. "Is Tom with a patient?"

"Yeah. What's up?" Linda answers. "You doin' okay? You want me to get him?"

"Tell him they think I have gangrene in my gallbladder. Just tell him," I shout. "Can you hear me?" The phone reception is breaking up as I come over the bridge. "Tell him I have *gangrene* in my *gallbladder* and I'm being admitted to the hospital right now." Some women would cry. That's not my way. I'll cry later.

In an hour, I'm lying in a pre-op bed.

It's hard to argue with gangrene.

I didn't even try.

❉   ❉   ❉

"They're going to try to do it through the scope," the nurse with bleached, spiked hair tells me briskly. I'm being brave and overly calm, asking all the right questions about the procedure. Though I've worked in hospitals for the last twenty years, I haven't been a patient in one since Mica was born. Zen and Orion, the two younger boys, were both delivered at home.

"Mrs. Harman?" asks an orderly with five-o'clock shadow who reminds me of someone in a gangster movie.

I nod.

"Ready for a little ride?" He smiles slyly, thinking he's cute.

I better get it together. I don't want to go into the OR for removal of a gallbladder and come out minus a kidney. I glance at my IV and shake my head to clear it. They may have already given me a sedative. "Yes," I say, holding out my arm with the plastic ID band on it, wanting him to double-check my name. He *did* say *Harman*, didn't he? Not *Hammond* or *Hartman?*

The orderly glances at the band without really reading it. "It's time to go. They're ready for you." As we roll away, I view the action in the large pre-op bay.

Nurses and doctors in blue scrubs transport patients back and forth, consulting with one another as I pass by. The professionals sound like they're speaking another language, and I feel like a character in someone's bad dream. We're inside an alien spaceship. They're the crew and I'm the stranger about to be probed. Then I'm moving fast down the hallway into the belly of the craft, and there's the smell of Betadine and antiseptic soap.

"Good luck," someone calls.

At the last minute my husband shows up, dressed in scrubs and wearing a green paper hat. He's not going to assist with the surgery; he's just here to make sure my soul doesn't float away in the middle of the operation. Tom's not an assertive guy, but if they're screwing up and letting my blood pressure drop, he'll say something. I think he'll say something . . . he won't let me die.

Tom jokes with the nurses, shakes hands with Dr. Jamison. I watch them discuss my case, leaning in toward each other. Then Tom comes over and touches my arm. "How you doing?" The OR is as comfortable to him as his study, the scrubs as comfortable as his pajamas. Not to me. As a midwife, my place is in the birthing room or the mother's bedroom. I enter the surgical suite, hesitantly, only when I assist with a C-section.

My husband's green eyes twinkle above the surgical mask as he bends over me. I want to touch his smooth tan cheek, and lifting my hand, I beckon him closer. "If I die," I whisper, pressing my forehead against his and not caring who hears us or what they may think, "I'll meet you in heaven."

I have tears in my eyes and I haven't loved him this much for a long while. Tom smiles indulgently. "Did you hear me?" I insist seriously. He's probably thinking it's the pre-op sedation making me goofy, but he pulls down his mask and kisses me.

I know Tom doesn't believe in heaven, but right now he needs to. This might be our last time together. "Promise?"

"Yeah," he says. "But you won't die."

They are rolling me into the OR now . . . "You never know," I say. "It could happen."

❖   ❖   ❖

I don't die. But three days later, I'm still in the hospital and I'm not doing well. I feel like shit. My blood oxygenation is poor. I'm short of breath, in too much pain, and my abdomen resembles an eight-month pregnancy.

I've decided I must have a pulmonary embolism, or maybe a massive hematoma under my diaphragm, but Dr. Jamison and my husband don't seem concerned. Maybe they're covering something up, trying to be reassuring.

I don't trust the nurses either. I'm an RN myself and I know I'm not getting the kind of care I would give. I time how long it takes them to answer the call light. Twenty minutes. I'd have been dead by then if I'd been having a stroke. I remind myself that there's a national nursing shortage and I should try not to be so demanding. They're probably attending to too many patients. That doesn't help. Now I'm really afraid.

Three days after the surgery, a massive transport aide with a triple chin comes to room 770 and says, "X-ray?" I didn't know I was getting an X-ray. I wonder what's up.

Across from the nurses' station, the orderly parks me; I'm on display while we wait for the elevator. He leans against the wall and salutes the ward secretary. Visitors' eyes linger, they're wondering what's wrong with me. I imagine how I must look; pale, disheveled. I haven't washed my hair for a week. Some of these people are my patients or families of patients that I have delivered. I pretend to be asleep, or maybe comatose. If I can't see them, maybe they won't see me.

❖   ❖   ❖

Late in the afternoon, when the sun slants in through the window, Dr. Jamison comes by to tell me that the X-ray showed I have an ileus. "It's unfortunate, but as you know it's not uncommon in prolonged or difficult surgeries. Your bowels have stopped moving and the gas in them is compressing your lungs, that's why you're short of breath and your oxygen saturation is so low." He looks rumpled and tired but takes time to ask about the huge bouquet of daisies and irises on the bedside table. "My sons," I explain, smiling fondly through the pain.

"If you can walk more," Jamison says, "you might increase the peristalsis of the bowels and get the gas moving. Otherwise, I can have the nurses put in a rectal tube." That sounds delightful.

I'm determined to get my paralyzed bowels in motion. After countless trips up and down the hall, pushing my IV pole and an oxygen tank, there are actual gas pains, spasms that almost double me over, and finally a fart. I stand in the carpeted corridor and let one rip, don't hold it back, and don't care if anyone hears. I fart some more, laughing.

That afternoon, since I'm feeling better, I decide to see what America's watching on TV. On *Oprah,* a couple discuss their history of domestic violence. The man is a cop. He got counseling.

I think of all the patients I've known who have lived with violent men. I think of my father and mother; their passion, their fights. A foreman at a trucking depot in the California Bay Area, my father commuted to Oakland from our subdivision in Walnut Creek. Every other Friday was payday, and that meant a stop at the pub. He came home five hours late, loaded and jolly, smelling of booze and cheap perfume. He sat at the piano with me, played "Chopsticks," and laughed. My mom, a substitute schoolteacher, as jealous as a cat, didn't say a word.

As soon as my brother and I were tucked in bed, the fight would begin. That's when I learned to be on guard, waiting for something bad to happen. The voices would rise and then something would smash against the wall: a piece of furniture, a dish, or sometimes my mother. I pulled a pillow over my head so I couldn't hear the swearing and the crying and things shattering. It didn't work. I could still hear.

In my hospital bed, flicking through the channels, I stop at a country-western video. It's about the passing of time and the shortness of life. I lie with tears running down my face. I'm weary of working so hard, of always worrying about patients and finances. How long have we been on this not-so-merry-go-round? The illness and the pain have burned a hole through me and cleaned something out. In the emptiness is hope. All day I am quiet inside myself. My life is a handful of sand. Whatever I have, however much sand is in there, it's all I've got left, all I'll ever have and it's leaking away, grain by grain, minute by minute.

❊   ❊   ❊

On the sixth day after admission, I'm finally discharged from the hospital. At home, I sit on the porch with a pink quilt tucked around me, thinking about my remaining grains of sand and what I'm going to do with them. All my thoughts about the IRS, the practice's debt, and my patients' problems have been washed away.

As I look out across our garden, I see that the beans are now four inches high. Below in the woods, redbud are blooming, pink against the dark trunks of maple. The intense West Virginia green almost hurts. Something catches my eye and I turn slowly, aware of my incisions.

Over the lake, a red-tailed hawk soars, and it seems that it's there for me personally, a sort of message. We are all here for one another, it says, winding through the tops of the trees. Gifts to one another. The green beans shooting through the soft earth, the redbuds, and the raptor soaring through the high branches, just glad to be here.

We are all here for one another and that is enough.

CHAPTER 5

ARAN

"It's going to be a *girl*. It *is* a girl, I mean," Aran bubbles when she
sees me walking down the clinic hall. She stands at the checkout
desk wearing skimpy jean shorts and a tight white T-shirt over her
rounding tummy. Her dark golden hair is clipped short, like a boy's.
Jimmy stands with her, his muscular left arm, tattooed with barbed
wire, wrapped protectively around her waist. He's let his hair grow,
and the messy red thatch sticks up at the top. Except for the multiple studs in Aran's ears, the girl has no other piercings, and no tattoo, I note. Unusual, these days.

"That's great," I say, admiring the ultrasound photo that Jimmy
reverently holds out. "Do you have a name picked out yet?"

"Not yet. We had to find out if it was a girl or a boy." Jimmy gently places the black-and-white photo in my hand as if it were a baby
bird. I inspect it, and the young father contributes, "You can see the
head, even the eyes and nose." He points them out with a thick
grubby finger.

"Are you taking good care of yourself, Aran? Taking your vitamins and eating okay?"

"She's doing good," Jimmy answers. "I make sure she gets fruits
and vegetables and meat every day." So far he's doing most of the
talking, and it's the most I've ever heard him say.

The young couple live in a thirty-foot trailer in Green Hills, out
on Route 26. I've seen the place from the bike trail along Wolf
Creek. It's clean inside but smells like mold, Trish told me. Still, it's
all they can afford, and Trish and Dan had to lend them money for

that. Jimmy has a job as an assistant bricklayer, and the young couple are doing better than might have been expected.

"Well, you look great, Aran. Doesn't she, Donna?" Donna, who sits at the checkout desk, glances up and smiles but keeps her fingers moving over her keyboard.

Today Aran's a rose in bloom. I return the ultrasound image to Jimmy. "It's a beautiful baby," I say. "Appears to be smart." I'm kidding, but the young couple inspect the photo like they're wondering how I can tell. Laughing, I give them both hugs then turn to go to my office. Halfway there, I glance back.

Aran and Jimmy are still leaning their elbows on the checkout counter, admiring their unborn baby. Maybe they'll be okay yet, I think, taking a breath.

It could happen.

Fall from Grace

At 2:15, I roll over in bed. I've been lying awake thinking about Aran and Trish, wondering how they are doing, and about the memo that came late yesterday from our accountant. I wish Mrs. Gorham had called or told us in person, but the woman acts as if coming to the office is an imposition, and she always writes letters or communicates by e-mail. Pittsburgh is three hours away. Maybe I expect too much. Tom would say so.

Our experience with accountants is limited. We've only had two. The first one, Bob Reed, was a total disaster. Bob, a short, balding ex-hippie with a ponytail, was affable and met with us in the conference room monthly, but he was incompetent. Since Tom and I had never been in business before, it took us two years to find out just how bad he was, and then another three months to fire him.

The new accountant seems to know what she's doing. I think she does, anyway; there's that air about her. And the woman has all kinds of awards and certificates on her office walls. There's a framed diploma from the University of Georgia and a plaque from the chamber of commerce. There's an article from the *Pittsburgh Post-Gazette* saying she's one of the rising businesswomen in the state, and a letter of appreciation from the ACLU for volunteer work.

I pull on my robe. In the bathroom, I find the jam jar of scotch and carry it into my study. This was the TV room a few years ago. I took it over for an office when our youngest boy went to college. The large white corner desk has space for my laptop and my printer, and there are two rows of cubbyholes for photographic equipment, prints, and negatives. There are two tall white bookshelves, a narrow daybed with a pink patchwork quilt, and a long bulletin board with snapshots of the boys.

There's a photo of Mica at ten kneeling next to Orion, who is three and carries his grandpa's lunch pail. There's Zen at six, with his new spiked haircut, all of them little blond boys. On the walls of the study and in every spare corner are prints, hand-thrown pottery, photography, and sculpture. After rummaging around in my brief-case, I pull out Gorham's letter and read it again.

Dear Dr. and Mrs. Harman,
Recent communication with Andy Bowlin at the regional IRS
office in Chicago has confirmed that the $21,000 adjustment
to your income tax for the previous two years is not an error.
I explained to Bowlin that the error was unintentional, but it
doesn't matter. Unless the back taxes are paid in full, in the
next ten days, there will be additional penalties. Please let me
know when you will be able to send the check.

I'm not sure why I needed to read the letter again. The meaning was plain the first three times. And the news is still bad. On my way to the porch, I pass through the kitchen, its white tile and whitewashed oak cabinets gleaming in the moonlight. I could say it isn't fair, or that the government's crooked. I could blame it on Bob Reed, but I just feel stupid.

Leaning against the porch rail, I tilt my head up. The stars are full out. How can my husband sleep? I resent it. Isn't he worried? I take a big gulp of scotch. Tomorrow I'll have to call Mrs. Gorham and tell her the truth, that we have no money. No doubt she assumes we have assets we can cash in, but we don't. We've no personal savings or surplus in the practice checking account, and no one to borrow from either, no sugar daddy anywhere.

Rebecca probably thinks that because Tom is a doctor, he's loaded, but he didn't go to med school until he was thirty, and he didn't finish his residency until he was thirty-eight. We're paying off his student loans at the same time we're putting the kids through college.

I take a deep breath and let it out slowly, remembering something I heard in my women's meditation group: "Let go and let God." I say it three times, trying to mean it. The sleep medicine has kicked in and I'm tired now. I leave the door to the porch open and crawl under the covers. Tom sleeps on blissfully, curled on his side with a pillow under his arm to support his bad shoulder.

I married an agnostic who has the faith in life of a born-again Christian. Sometimes I'd like to wake him up, make him wander the house with me. Make him stand on the shadowy deck, watching like a sea captain for icebergs ahead. If he were more concerned about office finances, the boys' futures, and the high cost of medical-malpractice insurance, I might worry less.

Other times, I'd like to wake him just to sit on the porch with me, sit in the dark looking out at the stars. We could share the mystery of unseen wild things moving through the woods, the sound of the water, the holy smell of the earth.

HEATHER

I am surprised to see Heather, my teenager pregnant with twins, added to the schedule late Friday afternoon. Her name appears in red, appropriately, on the computer printout: *Add-on: OB, bleeding.* I cringe. With the urgency of my gallbladder attack, the prolonged hospitalization, and three weeks of sick leave, I hadn't realized the young woman missed her last OB appointment. It's been over a month. At three o'clock, I knock apprehensively on the exam room door, not looking forward to the visit.

Before I have time to open my mouth, Mrs. Gresko starts in. "Well, she has *cramps* now too," the grandmother says. There's something about her tone that blames me. T.J.'s not present.

I settle myself on the stool. "Can you tell me how much bleeding you're having, Heather?" I want to ask why she'd skipped her last appointment. She could have seen Tom or one of the other nurse-practitioners while I was sick, but it doesn't really matter at this point.

Mrs. Gresko answers. "Not much now. It stopped for three weeks but there was *a lot* last night. There was blood all over the place." She still clutches the old white leather bag. Today the older woman is wearing a dark gray polyester jacket. I notice again how thin Heather is. Her little arms poke out of her lavender turtleneck, and I can see the nipples of her tiny breasts through the knit. Her skin is almost translucent.

"I'd like to see the sanitary pad with the blood on it," I say. The patient glances at her grandmother.

"She just changed in the bathroom. We didn't know you'd want it."

"Well, yes. It helps to see how much blood there is, and what color. I'll need to examine you too, Heather. Why don't you take off your bottoms while I go hunt for the pad." I hand her a folded white sheet.

"Do you have to check her? Can't you just do another ultra-sound?"

"No, now that she's having cramps, I really need to look inside her vagina and feel her cervix to see if it is starting to open. What Heather is experiencing . . ." I hate having to address the older woman when she isn't my patient. I swivel and direct my comments to Heather. "What you are experiencing, Heather, is called a *threatened miscarriage*. We always hope for the best in situations like this, but it's still important for me to see if anything's changed inside."

"Don't you think all this poking around could make her lose the babies? I don't really think it's a good idea." I see Mrs. Gresko's eyes narrow through the clear plastic cat's-eye frames.

Feeling like shouting, I force myself to answer calmly. "I'll be very gentle, Mrs. Gresko. What I'll be doing could never cause a miscarriage. Now, Heather," I say to the girl, who still hasn't spoken, "please undress while I hunt for your sanitary napkin. Just take off your pants and put this sheet over your lap. You don't need a whole gown. I'll put a disposable pad under your bottom to protect the exam table in case you bleed."

In the bathroom across the hall I put on gloves, fish through the stainless-steel trash can, and find the half-soaked mini pad under some paper towels. That's all I need. I tap on the exam room door and enter again. Heather has followed my instructions and is already lying with her feet in the footrests, her very thin legs spread apart passively. "I found it," I say. "It was right on top. Is that the most bleeding you've had?" I'm addressing Heather, with my back to the older woman, but Mrs. Gresko *still* answers.

"I told you it was *a lot more* last night. It's slowed down considerable." She has the upland accent of a family that's lived in Appalachia for generations. Without saying anything more, I sit down on the stool between Heather's legs. It's been a long week.

The amount of bright red blood pooled in Heather's vagina surprises me in light of what I've just seen on the pad. It takes three large cotton swabs to soak it all up. When I pull the swabs out, the vagina fills up with blood again. This isn't good. I glance up at Heather to see if she's hurting. It's impossible to tell. The girl stares intently at the ceiling.

"There *is* a fair amount of blood. Does this hurt?" I palpate the young woman's cervix and uterus.

"Does it hurt? Tell the doctor," says Mrs. Gresko. Heather hasn't had a chance to answer, but the old lady says it a second time, louder. "The doctor wants to know if it *hurts*," she shouts. Heather shakes her head no. When I pull off my gloves, I keep them low and quickly throw them into the trash to hide the red. It's a useless gesture. They know.

And I ignore the appellation of *doctor*. To remind Mrs. Gresko that I'm a *nurse-midwife* would only confuse things right now. Washing my hands, I notice my reflection in the small mirror next to the sink and straighten my dangling silver earrings. I look older today, and my head hurts. Maybe I look older because I'm so tired. I pull back my shoulders, run both hands through my hair, and smooth my aqua silk shirt, then I sit back on the stool.

"Well, there's good news and there's bad," I start off. "I really don't like the appearance of all that blood. It's more than I expected."

"I told you there was a lot," says Grandma.

I nod. "Still, the cervix is closed. That's a good sign. We need to do another ultrasound to check the fetal heart tones."

"That's what we came for," says Mrs. Gresko.

"Well, that comes next. I need to go see if the ultrasound room is empty."

As I round the corner, I get lucky. "Hey, am I glad to see *you*," I say, coming up behind Tom. He's squatting down in his office, searching for something on the bottom shelf of his bookcase. He's wearing light blue scrubs that hang low on his hips. His royal blue scrub cap is tied at the back of his head. Grinning, he pulls me toward him, trying to get his mouth on my neck. I struggle a little. *Now I don't feel so old!*

"Come on. Be serious." I laugh, trying to straighten my collar. "Let's have a little professionalism around here!"

"What's up?" He lets go and flops down in his leather chair.

"You remember Heather? The young woman with twins?"

"Yeah? They're taking my patient into the OR any minute, I have to go back to the hospital." He knows I'm going to ask him for something.

"Well, she called with increased bleeding. The nurse had her come in, and there's *a lot* of blood, not just a little. I was surprised. Could you do another ultrasound?"

He's standing up. "Come on. Let's go. Is she in there?"

"No, I'll get her. She's already undressed. You set up."

I run back to the exam room and explain to the patient that if we hurry we can do the ultrasound right now. Trying not to be rude, I wrap a sheet around Heather and rush both women down the hall to the corner exam room, where Dr. Harman is waiting. For the first time, I see that the older lady limps. I'd noticed her dark swollen legs before. She's a setup for blood clots.

In contrast to the last time, this visit is cheerless. Tom explains that twin number one no longer has a heartbeat. The *threatened* miscarriage had turned into an *actual* miscarriage, complicated by the presence of a remaining live fetus.

"There's not really anything we can do now but watch and wait. The other twin might still make it," he tells the young woman and her grandmother. Then his pager goes off. "I'm sorry, I have to go. They have a patient ready for me in the operating room." He rests a hand on Heather's shoulder. "I'm sorry," he says again. Then he pats her arm, nods at Grandma, and leaves.

I slowly turn up the lights with the rheostat, then sit on the exam stool. In the dark, I'd thought Heather showed no emotion and I'd wondered if she even understood, but now I see her wipe her eyes with the tips of her fingers. For once, Mrs. Gresko is quiet. She adjusts the strap of her white leather bag, fiddling with the gold buckle.

"I'm sorry too. I was hoping both babies would make it. Even with all that blood, I thought they might." The two women are silent. "Do you understand what Dr. Harman said, Heather, Mrs. Gresko? One baby has died. The fetus closer to the opening is still alive, but it's at risk. If the bleeding gets too heavy, you may have to have a D and C to take both babies out, but there's no way to take out the one that's dead without hurting the live baby. Eventually your body will absorb it. We'll have to watch carefully for infection, of course. We can't take a chance on your health or your ability to have more children."

Heather clears the tears from her throat. "I don't understand why it happened." It's the first time today the girl has pronounced a full sentence, and her beautiful low voice still surprises me. I scoot up closer on the rolling exam stool and touch Heather's knee, expecting her to pull away, but she doesn't. She stares at my lined, freckled hand, which looks almost as old as Mrs. Gresko's. I stare at it too. That's what washing your hands at the exam room sink before and after each patient will do. I should use more lotion.

Mrs. Gresko is probably not even near seventy, she just looks it. Hard life in the mountains, cigarettes, and poor nutrition make women age prematurely. I wonder whether Mrs. Gresko raised Heather or if she's just standing in for Heather's working mom, but I don't want to ask.

"We hardly ever understand why this happens," I answer carefully. "Something just wasn't forming right. There's nothing you or anyone did to cause the miscarriage and there's nothing we can do to make it stop. It's just nature's way of insuring that most of the babies that *are* born are perfect."

Heather nods and wipes her eyes again.

"So nothing could have been done, even if we'd come to see you earlier? No medicine or anything? There's *nothing* you could have done?" Mrs. Gresko asks.

I shake my head no. "Nothing but wait and hope."

The grandmother raises her eyebrows and lets out a long tired breath.

Reprieve

Lying in bed tonight, I feel a sense of relief, despite everything. Outside, through the open screen door, a rare loon laughs on Hope Lake. Maybe Gorham isn't so bad. When I'd gone up to Pittsburgh to explain there was no way we could pay the IRS in a lump sum, she'd looked up from her desk, which was cluttered with papers, books, and pencils, twisted a strand of her red hair, the gold bangles on her wrists catching the light, and suggested we get another bank loan.

"It's done all the time," she told me. "They use the assets of the practice as collateral. Your ultrasound machine would cover the loan." This evening after work, Tom and I'd signed the promissory note for twenty-one thousand dollars and mailed the check to our accountant.

How long ago was it that we had no debts? I calculate back. On the communal farm, we paid cash for everything. We didn't need much, just gas for the truck, peanut butter, rice, whole wheat flour, canola oil, and beans. We grew all the rest.

When we went back to nursing and medical school, we got student loans, then a few credit cards. When Tom got out of residency and joined the faculty at the university hospital, we took out a loan for our first house, and a few years later borrowed more for the cottage on the island in Lake Erie. I picture the two-story yellow farmhouse that sits on the rocky waterfront, the expanse of lawn and the willow trees, the red-roofed barn. It was worth it.

We started our private practice at Community Hospital with a loan from the bank; then we borrowed for the ultrasound machine, got money to set up our new partner, Dr. Burrows, in practice, took a loan for the laser equipment, and now this, another twenty-one thousand. I grimace. It adds up. But by the end of the week, the sword of the IRS will no longer hang over our heads, and we can make payroll. Tonight, the waters of Lake Hope lie quiet, lapping the shore.

TRISH

I haven't seen Trish for days, I've been so preoccupied with our own financial problems, and then I spot her trudging across the employee parking lot after work. "Trish!" I call out. "Hey, wait up." She turns slowly, tucking her sandy blond hair behind her ear.

"How are things?"

"Oh, up and down. You know. My life's such a drama." Trish laughs at herself.

"What's happening? I haven't seen Aran since we transferred her to the teen OB clinic at the university hospital. She doin' okay?" We walk across the blacktop together.

"Jimmy got laid off after he had a fight with one of the other workers but found a new job doing landscaping. Then he didn't like his boss and quit. Aran moved home again this weekend. It's the third time she's come back. She says she's *through* with him now. To tell you the truth, I hope so. This stress is killing me."

I groan sympathetically. Sometimes I don't know how Trish stands these ups and downs, ins and outs.

"How's Dan doing?"

"Oh, you can guess. He's just withdrawing from the situation, trying to maintain. He's getting stomachaches and has started smoking again. I'm getting stomachaches too, right here." She puts the palm of her hand below her heart. "Acid maybe, something cold and bitter like rust. I don't know. A premonition, mother's intuition, maybe. I feel like I should be doing something to help Aran, but she won't let me." Trish stops to unlock her car. "Sorry—I have to hurry. I have an appointment. I'm going to have my hair highlighted. It's the first time." She laughs again. "The gray's coming in fast and I'm only thirty-five!"

Twenty minutes later I'm at the Veterans Memorial Park in bike shorts. Tom hands me my helmet and gloves, and without more than a few words we hit the trail. We pedal along the Jefferson River, past the dam, where the water churns gray and a few logs bob up and down in the foam. Here Asian men fish for bass and the occasional trout. These are university students from China, I imagine, enjoying the sunshine and a social pastime that reminds them of home. We pass the kids' jungle gyms and slides, where I nearly always see a mother with a child I'd delivered, now a toddler in a stroller. Sometimes I stop to talk, but today I pedal on.

We roll through successive waves of fragrance where honeysuckle vines grow along the riverbank. Pink phlox and blue chicory bend in the wind. Tom stops and points out an indigo bunting on a low sumac bush.

Trish's hair is turning gray, and mine is more than half silver, but on the bike trail I'm still twenty-five.

Harvest Song

The radishes and sugar peas are ready to harvest. Today I'm picking the peas by the handful and throwing them into a basket, grabbing the thin pods, my back bent over, then pulling the radishes up by their veined green leaves and washing them under the hose. This could take hours, and I'm not in the mood. I love planting and seeing things grow, but I plant too much and then have to tend it. When we lived on the farm, we preserved hundreds of jars of produce, but harvesting in those days was fun.

Six or eight of us and Mica would gather in the big log house, the men mostly bearded and sweaty, the women in shorts or long skirts with no bras. We'd sit on homemade oak benches around a long wooden table, chopping tomatoes or stringing beans. Sometimes we'd sing while we worked. Spirituals would ring out through the open windows in perfect four-part harmony. Now I pick peas alone, not as enjoyable, but still good . . . good to grow your own food. Roscoe, our trusty basset-beagle, follows me along the rows, thinking I might find something she can eat. Despite the name, Roscoe's a female. Zen got her when he was fourteen. Our youngest son had always wanted a dog named after Rosco P. Coltrane, the sheriff in the old TV show *The Dukes of Hazzard*. He didn't care if it was a female.

The dry clots of dirt hurt my bare feet, and the sun warms my back. Nearly everyone in West Virginia has a vegetable plot. The garden might be only one or two tomato plants out on the porch, or acres of potatoes and corn. If they don't have their own, they get produce from the brothers who still live on the family places in Big Sulphur Springs or Clover Gap.

Homegrown vegetables, deer meat, and trout are the soul food of Appalachia. It's the Little Debbie Devil Cremes at the 7-Eleven, the fried chicken, and the bacon grease on the green beans that give us one of the highest rates of obesity in the nation.

On the commune we did everything by Rodale's *Encyclopedia of Organic Gardening*. "Rotate your crops from year to year to renew the nitrogen." "Never place zucchini next to yellow squash; they'll cross-pollinate." "Don't weed beans when they're wet, you'll spread leaf wilt." Lately, I just garden when I have the time and plunk the plants where there's space. What I put in the ground doesn't always flourish. I tend my plants like I tended my kids. The boys got abundant love, but maybe not the pruning and direction they needed. I fear my children are ill prepared for this world. They grew up like wildflowers, sometimes like weeds.

I stand up from my labors in the garden and stretch my back, looking out across the clearing to the gazebo. Let's face it: Tom and I, too, are ill prepared for this world.

CHAPTER 6

HEATHER

"Dr. Harman," Tom says, flipping open the cell phone he keeps on the small bedside table. I elbow myself up in the dark to squint at the red numerals on the alarm clock. Shit. I might have slept through the night if he hadn't been paged. It's 3:00 a.m.

"How much is she bleeding?" my husband asks. I turn on the green and white stained-glass dresser lamp.

"I'll be right in. Will you call the nursing supervisor, alert the OR, and have her typed and crossed for two units?" He's already on his way to the closet, where a pile of blue scrubs are stacked on a shelf.

"What's up?"

"Patient hemorrhaging. Miscarriage." He's a man of few words.

"Heather?" I know the answer.

"Yeah, the girl with twins." He's tying his running shoes. "See you in a few hours." Tom flicks off the light, then closes the door. I lie awake, flooded with adrenaline, as I always am when the phone rings at night.

Throwing back the covers, I pad through the house. On the porch, I pull up a deck chair, take a sip of my bitter sleep medicine, and rest my chin on the rail. In three hours my alarm will go off. There's no sound but the rain and the trucks on the highway a mile away.

Tom will be driving fast. In the middle of the night, it's thirteen minutes to Community Hospital, longer during the day. We know exactly how fast we can get there after all the years of doing obstetrics.

He streaks through the traffic light near the Mountain Plaza and avoids the Torrington business district, where the winding streets that lead to the Jefferson River slow you down. Now he pulls into the ER parking lot and clicks his remote lock at the Toyota. He steps calmly out of the elevator into the harsh light of the fifth-floor pre-op bay. I see Heather's white face, wet with tears, when she sees him.

Calling

Some people are born to be midwives. I think about that. Going back to school took work, sacrifice, and student loans, but I decided to go after my first delivery, which I did by accident.

Laura, dressed in denim coveralls and about seven months pregnant, seeks me out at the Growing Tree Whole Foods Co-op. "I want to have my baby naturally, can you help me with the breathing?" she says, swinging her long blond braid back over her shoulder. "I heard you had Mica that way. Will you help me?"

We meet four times in the back room of the natural-food store that our commune started; it's located across the street from the courthouse in Spencer. Sitting behind a row of five-gallon buckets of peanut butter, barrels of whole wheat flour, and sacks of oats and pinto beans, we go over deep breathing, shallow breathing, staying centered, and trusting your body. I had taught Lamaze classes and read a few books. I'd attended two hospital deliveries as a labor coach, and I'd had one baby myself. That was the extent of my knowledge. It made me a local expert.

"The breathing doesn't really take away the pain. It just gives you something to do when you want to run away, which you can't do anyway, so why even try!" I tell her. Laura laughs.

"You can hum or count backward. It all works the same." I show her some tricks of positioning, some techniques for massage.

Three weeks before her due date, Laura and her husband, Lou, ask Tom and me to come over for dinner and one last childbirth class. They live in a large converted barn in relative luxury, four couples and three kids under seven.

On Saturday we drive down the rutted dirt road into their hollow. On either side of the narrow lane, redbud and dogwood are blooming, everything's alive and expanding. The barn, a huge, sturdy, insulated two-story structure, comes into view. I'm impressed when Lou gives us a tour. Each family has its own space in the loft. The common areas are downstairs: kitchen, living room, and library. The commune even boasts an indoor commode and hot running water. After dark, when a spring snowstorm comes up, we decide to sleep over rather than get the jeep stuck in the mud. Tom, Mica, and I are shown to an empty bedroom, and after a luxurious hot shower, we settle down for the night.

Around three I hear rustling, low voices, and footsteps back and forth to the john. Maybe one of the commune's toddlers is sick . . . Tom sleeps through it all. At four in the morning, Star comes to our door. "Can you come, Patsy? Please! Something is happening."

I pull on my jeans and turtleneck and follow the woman up wooden stairs. Star wears a long paisley skirt and has disheveled golden hair down to her waist. She looks as if she's been up all night. "At first it just seemed like a backache," she whispers. "But it's got to be more than that. I've never had a kid, so what do I know? Laura's been up most of the night. Now she's started to puke and there's blood down her legs."

The small woman pads down the hall on her calloused bare feet and leads me up narrow wooden steps. We stop at the door to a bedroom illuminated by dozens of candles. Pachelbel's *Canon* plays low on the stereo. On a mattress on the floor, Laura crawls naked, moaning and swinging her head.

Lou kneels beside her in shorts and a tie-dyed shirt, massaging her back. His long ponytail droops over his shoulder. "It's coming, Patsy! I don't know what to do. We planned a home birth and I was supposed to catch but I can't. I just can't . . ." His face is as white as the bedsheets. "*You* have to do it," he says to me.

I go very still. *Pregnant woman . . . almost full term . . . moaning . . . blood . . . muddy roads . . . hospital two hours away.* That's what I'm thinking. Then there's a pop, Laura groans, and a gush of clear fluid squirts out of her vagina. "Go get Tom, Star, he's hard to wake up. You'll have to shake him—and get the birth kit. You have something prepared, don't you, Lou, some supplies?" The man looks around wildly.

"Top drawer—bureau," Laura snaps between moans. "My back hurts so bad. Damn! I have to push, but when I do it only hurts worse." She lets out a wail and starts shaking. So much for childbirth breathing. "Get a grip, Laura," I tell her. "Yelling is not gonna help, and it scares the baby." I don't know where I came up with that line, but it works. I've used it a hundred times with women in labor since then. She shuts up.

Then Tom steps into the room with Star and takes in the situation at a glance. "Where's the birth stuff?"

"Inside the chest. I need some gloves. She's gotta push."

Something is bulging between Laura's legs as she wags her butt back and forth, and I haven't even washed my hands. Tom pulls a paper sack out of the drawer and finds a box of exam gloves. They aren't sterile, but neither is anything else, and they'll have to do.

"It's almost over, Laura. I'm going to touch you. Don't move around." I part her labia and am startled to find a head covered with dark wet hair, about the size of a large apple.

Laura moans again. "I got to get this fucking baby out of there. It's killing me." She growls like something coming out of the earth, and the head moves a quarter inch into my hands.

"What's in the bag besides gloves, Tom? Shoe strings, scissors?" Tom isn't a paramedic or a doc. He hasn't even thought of being one yet. He's a bearded hippie beekeeper with the shoulders and arms of a carpenter and the soul of a string bass player.

"Scissors in a plastic baggie with shoelaces. Some gauze and a blue infant suction thing. There are some worry beads, a baby blanket, and a laminated picture of Krishna." He drops the beads in the drawer and hands Lou the picture of Krishna. The medical supplies he lays out on a pink flannel baby blanket, and then he puts on gloves himself.

"I don't suppose you could roll over?" I ask Laura between her contractions. She's still rocking back and forth on her knees. "Lay on your back?"

"Oh, shit," she says, and she's right. As the baby slides down the birth canal, some BM moves through the rectum and out of the way. Tom takes some gauze and wipes it up. Everything is moving fast now, but the baby's head doesn't flex. I know from the drawings in the emergency-childbirth manual that you should *keep the head flexed,* but this baby's upside down with its chin tucked under the pubic bone, and I haven't a clue what to do so I just hold on and put my hands around the head like a crown.

"Breathe it out now," I say with authority. "Breathe it out slowly." Laura breathes. "Now pant!" A baby's face is emerging from between Laura's legs, scrunched and blue, looking up at the ceiling.

Tom reaches over and suctions the mouth like he's done this before. "It's trying to suck on the bulb," he says, laughing. "Good sign." Then the whole wet mass swivels and shoots out onto the bed. I scoop it up. The infant's still dangling from the umbilical cord.

"A baby!" the father yells, then slumps into the fetal position. The newborn screams.

Laura laughs. "That wasn't so bad!" Women always say that when it's all over. I look between the infant's wet legs.

"It's a girl."

"I told you!" says Lou, raising his head.

After we tie off the cord and dry the infant, I hand the baby to her mother. The placenta slips out easily a minute later. Lou pulls himself together, and the three of them squirm to the head of the bed, where it's still dry. I throw a blanket across them, and the candlelight shines on their faces.

Behind Star, in the doorway, stands the rest of the commune. Three men and two women in various states of dress or undress, two sleepy toddlers, and one baby, who's being held by his mother and sucking on a breast. Mica sleeps through it all.

No one says anything, not even the kids, not a word. Pachelbel still plays on the stereo, music of holiness . . . Tom and I just kneel on the bed in the wet amniotic fluid.

Baptized.

SHIANA

"I think I might have herpes," the young coffee-skinned woman bursts out and then begins to sob. She doesn't just leak tears. She floods. There's no way to ask what's going on, or why she thinks she has an infection. *"The son of a bitch,* I'll never forgive him."

When a woman says she has herpes, it's usually fifty-fifty; half the time it's herpes, half the time it's something else. Sometimes it's a painful yeast infection, a boil, or an abrasion after sex. Sometimes it's a bump in the mucosa that's been there all along but the patient has just noticed it . . . and sometimes it's herpes.

We deal with alphabet soup nowadays. HSV (herpes simplex virus), HPV (human papillomavirus), HIV (human immunodeficiency virus). They're all sexually transmitted. Only one of them can directly kill you. The rest are just uncomfortable and with you for life.

I sit and wait for Shiana's tears to stop so I can ask her why she thinks she has herpes.

She's wearing the regulation thin cotton gown, sitting on the end of the exam table, with her dark hair pulled back under the pink baseball cap. I roll my stool up and hand her the tissues.

Shiana wipes her face, glances at me, then starts crying again. I pat the girl's knee and say something soothing. "It's okay now, sweetie. It's okay, hon. Tell me what's happening."

The young woman wipes her face and takes a deep breath.

"Why do you think you have herpes? What's going on?" I ask again softly.

Shiana swallows hard and lets out some air. Then her almond eyes water and it seems for a minute like I'm losing her again. I reach out and take the young woman's hand. "Let me take a look. Let's see what's going on down there. Maybe we can do cultures to find out for sure. Sometimes I can tell by examining you." I want to cut to the chase, but the girl doesn't lie back or put her feet in the footrests.

"Do you remember me?" Shiana asks. "I know you meet a lot of patients . . . I'm the girl with the condom. The blue one."

"I remember."

"Well, it's been downhill since I saw you. I got your nurse's call about the positive chlamydia test and I took the antibiotics like you told me, but then I got a yeast infection." She's talking fast now. Trying to get it all out. "I'd never had one before, but they said it was common after taking antibiotics . . . Now I'm all swollen and have little blisters down there. I checked on the Internet and I don't know what else it could be. It has to be herpes."

She starts leaking tears again, but before she gets too far, I say, "Shiana, stop now. I need your cooperation. I want you to lie down. I can usually tell by looking, but if I can't, I'll send cultures to the lab. Have you been sick with a fever or had any difficulty peeing?"

"It burns awful. It hurts so bad that I try not to pee. All I did yesterday was stay in bed. I didn't even tell my roommate what was wrong. I'm so ashamed."

I spread the young woman's outer labia with my gloved fingers. I don't need cultures, but I'll get them anyway. Along the right side are a row of white ulcers, tiny moist craters. There's no question.

"It's herpes," I say. "I was hoping it wasn't." Shiana puts her arm over her eyes and begins to sob again, this time silently, but her whole body shakes. It's hard to tell if it's sadness or anger.

"Shiana, I know you're upset, but I want you to sit up and listen to me. I'm going to tell you what we need to do." Shiana wipes her face and sits up, her hands folded in her lap on the blue exam gown, like a schoolgirl in the principal's office. She blows her nose on the tissues I give her.

"The first thing is, I'm going to give you medicine to make the sores go away. I want you to stay on the pills for two weeks. I'll get you something for the pain, and you'll probably need to take a few days off school. I know you're upset, but this isn't the end of the world." Shiana squints like she doesn't believe me. "No, really. I see two or three women a week with herpes." This is a lie, but sometimes I exaggerate to make the patients feel better. Really it's more like two or three cases a month.

"Will the medicine cure it?"

"No, it can't, but it can control the virus and dry up the sores. I had a herpes outbreak once." Shiana stops crying, paying close attention now, her brown eyes still shining with tears.

"*You?*"

"Yeah. I was about your age, nineteen or twenty. We didn't know about chlamydia then, or herpes, or HIV. This was back in the hippie days."

Shiana watches me, no doubt picturing the young Patsy Harman with hair to her waist, a long calico skirt, and maybe a flower behind her ear, like girls on a PBS special about the protest days. She wouldn't be far off.

"I had it much worse than you, and there weren't any antiviral medicines. I was at home on spring break and I got sores all over down there, and in my mouth too." For a second, I wonder if I'm being too graphic. I can't picture Tom or any other health-care provider telling a patient something like this, but I continue. Maybe it will help Shiana to know that someone else has been through this.

"It stung so bad when I had to go to the bathroom, I had to stand up in the tub to urinate."

"That's what I did too." The girl smiles. "I stood in the shower and tried to get the water to spray on me while I was peeing. It didn't help much."

I write my patient a script for acyclovir ointment and tablets and give her a pamphlet on living with herpes. "In seven days I'll see you again and we can discuss how you'll need to protect yourself and any future partners."

Shiana regards me, startled. I can tell she hadn't thought about what she would tell a new boyfriend. She's dressed now in a loose gray Torrington State University sweat suit. For a minute, I think of taking her to my home. The sweet young woman could use some mothering. But I resist. Like most professionals, I try to draw a line between my relationships with patients and my personal life. Though I've thought of doing it many times, I don't take them home.

"Well, I won't be telling *any* partners. I'm planning on being celibate from now on," the girl says, and the tears well up. This time there's no smile.

I give her a hug. I've said that myself. More than once.

KASMAR

Straightening the stethoscope around my neck, I take a deep breath and then open the door. "Hi, Kasmar." I reach out my hand, hoping I won't regret my decision to help her become a man. There are so many things I haven't thought out. Will the nurses object and refuse to give her the injections of testosterone? Will the other patients be offended to see someone who appears to be a man sitting in the waiting room?

The tall, thin woman sits in the guest chair; she's wearing neatly pressed gray slacks with a light green checkered shirt, the long sleeves rolled up. This time her dark hair is cropped even shorter and the neck shaved; no makeup, no earrings or jewelry, only a large square-faced gold watch with a leather band. Kasmar looks at me expectantly.

"So, how are you today?" I ask. It's been more than a month since her last visit.

"Fine, thank you." Kasmar shifts her ankle up on her knee and leans forward, waiting.

"Well, I suppose you're wondering what we've decided, so I might as well get to the point."

Kasmar watches my face.

"Dr. Harman and I had a discussion. We've decided that though your request is out of the ordinary, it's something that we can help you with."

She swallows hard, relief in her blue eyes.

I go on. "We'll help you so long as the testosterone injections aren't hurting your health. If we start to feel the situation is out of our league or requiring too much time, we reserve the right to stop treatment. I've also drawn up a consent form for you to sign in which you acknowledge that there are possible side effects to the—" I haven't finished my sentence but Kasmar is reaching for the heavy black ballpoint clipped in her front shirt pocket.

"Thanks so much," she says, signing the document after glancing over it, her tanned, freckled face flushed with excitement. "This is great." She's grinning from ear to ear. "This is just great."

I go over the potential side effects again. "Most of them are minor and reversible, like acne, cessation of periods, headaches, mood change, and masculinization." We both smile at that. "But some might be *irreversible*, like hair loss, liver problems, hypertension, or elevated cholesterol." Kasmar nods. She knows all this. Then I write the first script for the testosterone injections. Kasmar will pick up the syringe at the pharmacy and bring it to the clinic every two weeks.

If the patient had been born with a deformity, some error of nature such as a cleft lip or a clubfoot, someone would help her. To Kasmar, her female body is just as much of a mistake.

Kasmar stands, reaches for my hand, and pumps it firmly, still beaming. "This is great. Just great," she says again.

Her voice is already a few notes lower.

HOLLY

On sunny summer days, everyone at the clinic, from Dr. Tom to Junie, our junior secretary, is eager to go home early. Sometimes we close at four, but not often. We find ourselves dreaming of what we could be doing outside: working in the garden, biking, swimming, or just reading a book out on the porch.

Today's that kind of day. It's lunch break, and having finished my charting, I gaze for a minute out the window at the billowy white clouds being swept across the blue sky. Last night was that kind of night too! I smile, remembering.

Tom and I had our first skinny dip of the season. The air was warm, the dark waters of Hope Lake a little cold, just enough to make you holler when you dove in, although two minutes later you were swimming around and saying, "This is great!" "Not too bad." "Actually pretty warm."

In the cove below the house, skinny-dipping has the added benefit of being a little risky. How would it look if a well-known middle-aged physician and his wife were caught naked in the spotlight of a motor boat?

We swam on our backs, looking up at the stars. Dark sky, no moon yet. We dog-paddled into the streaks of silver and gold that floated over the black water from the cottages on the other side of the cove. We swam together, our bare bodies wrapped around each other. We played like little kids, grabbing each other's private parts. Well, I grabbed his, anyway, and joked about a snapping turtle.

There's a tap at my door, and I snap back to the here and now. "Your first patient is ready, chickie," says Celeste, my nurse for the afternoon, handing me a yellow chart. "Time to go back to work. Sure would be nice to leave early today." I know what she's really saying: *Try to keep up so we can leave on time, maybe even early.* I'll try. I always *try*.

I knock my usual greeting—*dum-de-dum-dum*—and enter exam room 1.

"Do you think this microdermabrasion would do me any good?" Holly Knight asks before I even get through the door. She inspects her face in the small gold-framed mirror mounted in the dressing corner.

"I think it does *good* for everyone. For you, it would take off the dry skin and some of the fine wrinkles. It would fade the sun damage." I turn Holly's face to the light. "It would clean out the pores . . . And it *feels* great."

It strikes me as odd that I, an ex-hippie who rarely wears makeup, promote medical cosmetic microdermabrasion, but I've come to feel that if a person can afford it, she should have her interest encouraged. In Torrington, because of the university, there are plenty of female professionals who travel, who read. They're curious how such procedures can help them.

Women don't do enough nice things for themselves. They give to their kids, their husbands, their parents and families. Sometimes they volunteer in the community or at church, but they rarely give to themselves. Whenever a patient signs up for a package, it's a celebration for us all.

I pat Holly on the back. "You should try it. Abby, our nurse, does a facial massage afterward and she has soft music playing. Every time I get one I think, *I've got to take better care of myself.* It makes me want to eat healthier, to exercise, to begin doing yoga again. We started doing the treatments when we stopped delivering babies. It helps pay the bills, and it's fun to help women feel good."

Holly sits down in the guest chair. Today she's dressed in a sleeveless aqua tunic, linen cropped pants, and taupe slides. Her highlighted hair is held back with a clip, but there are circles under her eyes and she looks tired.

I wonder how her daughter, Nora, is doing but hate bringing it up. The last I'd heard, she was in the ICU for bulimia. "So, how you been?" I start out, opening the chart.

"Oh, not too bad." Holly slides down in her chair with her long legs stretched out. "I think I need to change my antidepressant, though. It's not working. I'm so cranky I can hardly stand myself. Maybe I just need to increase the dose." She looks at me.

"Are you on it for perimenopausal symptoms, stress, anxiety, or depression?"

Holly laughs. "All of the above." That's what I like about this woman. She isn't a whiner, and except when it comes to her issues around her daughter, she can make fun of herself. We're quiet for a moment.

"So, how are you doing with your hormone replacement? Do you have enough to get you through till your annual gyn visit?"

"Yeah, I'm okay. I stopped taking the medication for a while. Did I tell you? But I went back. I started hot flashing and sweating all day. I thought I could make it naturally, but I can't and I don't know how some women do. I feel like a wimp." She waits for reassurance.

"We're all different, that's for sure. Some women's menopausal symptoms aren't that bad, others are so affected they can't work, they can't sleep, they can't make love, they can't remember their own kids' names." We laugh, both knowing how *that* is.

I laugh a lot with my patients. I joke with them about constipation. I kid about periods. We poke fun at aging, at looking in the mirror and seeing our mothers looking back at us. "We're being silly," I say when our laughter gets too loud, but sometimes if you don't laugh you might cry.

I open Holly's chart to her history. "You have no personal or family experience of breast cancer or early strokes, so the risk, if there is one, is worth the improvement in the quality of your life. You know what Dr. Harman says about hormone replacement, don't you?" Holly shakes her head no. "There's a risk in getting in a car and going across town too, but that doesn't mean you stay home." I raise my eyebrows to make the point. Holly grins.

"I always feel better when I come to see you, Patsy. I feel *almost* normal, like you understand."

I smile and nod. We are all *almost* normal. "So how's your stress level? Stress makes hot flashes worse, you know."

"Better, I guess. Nora's home from the treatment center and taking classes at State. I think she's still vomiting but she's holding her own. I told you she went to Atlanta to a treatment center for a month, didn't I?"

I shake my head no. "Did it help?"

Holly continues. "It seemed to at first, but then she comes home and starts puking again. My husband tells me I can't save her. I know he's right. She has to save herself." The patient's husband is the vice president of First Mountain State Bank. I met him once at a United Way fund-raiser.

"Why does she do it? The vomiting. Is it insecurity? Is it pressure at school?" I lean back against the cool white wall, wanting to understand. I wish I could take Holly home with me and have tea. We'd sit in my living room with our feet on the coffee table and talk about our kids and where we'd gone wrong. We'd eat brownies and maybe drink Stress Relief tea. I'd get out the pictures of Mica and Orion and Zen, and she'd open her wallet and show me her boys and Nora.

"I don't know why she vomits. I don't even think *she* knows anymore. It started when she was in junior high school. Now she can't stop. We have a new counselor but I'm afraid to hope. It's been such a struggle. I try to be optimistic, but if she gets really sick again I'm clueless what we'll do next, where we'll go.

"Thank God we have health insurance. I don't know what people do who don't have coverage. Do you know how much it costs to stay at a center for eating disorders? Fifteen hundred a day." Holly widens her eyes, waiting for my reaction. She gets what she expected.

"Fifteen hundred *a day?*" I know I heard right, but I can't comprehend it. "That's *forty-five thousand* for a month. Did you look around? Is that the going rate? Forty-five thousand!"

"Of course I did. Are you kidding? I got on the Internet to investigate and called every program. And there's only a limited amount of reimbursement on most health insurance plans for mental health, anyway. Did you know that?" the mother continues. "When you use it up, you're done, there's no more. Some of the centers will give you a break if you don't have coverage, but there's so much demand and so many young women with bulimia and anorexia. What would you do if she was your child? Mortgage your house? What would you do?" Her voice breaks. "You couldn't let your own daughter starve."

I nod. I know the passion mothers have for their children, and I wonder where Tom and I would get that kind of money if one of our kids were dying and we didn't have insurance. I would sell everything we own for one of my boys. You give birth to them in pain. You nurse them at your breast. You hold them at your heart forever.

I write Holly a script for her increased dose of antidepressants, give her a couple months' worth of samples of hormone replacement, then hold out a pamphlet on coping with stress. "Maybe this will help," I say, smiling. We both know it won't. I put my arms around Holly, saying a silent prayer for her daughter. Sometimes the mother needs mothering. We're almost the same height, both tall, big, capable women. Both little girls.

Shame

Okay, I'm ashamed about the alcohol . . . but not about the insomnia. I know from talking to so many women that half of them don't sleep well either. I've come to think of the sleeplessness as a disability, something I just have to live with. I never tell my patients about my sleep medicine. I don't tell Holly or Trish or Nila. I don't know why.

Okay, I do know. It's the shame of not being able to turn off my thoughts, of using a drug that, though legal, when taken too long and in excess can destroy your liver and maybe your mind.

I'm a midwife. When I discuss sleep problems with my patients, I talk about herbal teas, relaxed deep breathing, leaving their troubles out of the bedroom. Those things don't work for me. I doubt they work for them. Sometimes I prescribe pills for my patients or refer them to the sleep clinic. I went there myself a few years ago, but it was a waste. And I've tried sleeping pills too. I've never found one that both works and doesn't make me too groggy in the morning.

I used to believe my wakefulness came from delivering babies. For almost twenty years I was on call, and the phone would ring in the night. Someone would be in labor or in some kind of trouble. Sometimes I would lie awake just waiting for the telephone to ring or the pager to go off.

In reality, the wakefulness started long before, in a small tract house in California where I would lie listening to my parents shouting and to furniture crashing. It was my mama screaming, my father throwing things. I was eight or nine then, huddled in a twin bed in a small bedroom I shared with my brother. My bed was against the wall, his by the window. I used to wonder if I could get him out that window if I had to.

CHAPTER 7

HEATHER

I lean on the lab counter, skimming my last progress note. My teenage patient, Heather Moffett, has returned to the clinic. It's a follow-up visit for the emergency D & C of her twins. I dread the visit, expecting to be grilled by the stern grandmother, Mrs. Gresko, and perhaps also by the angry young man, T.J.

I'm surprised to find only Heather in the room, sitting in the visitor's chair and reading *Vogue*. She's dressed in worn blue jeans with a striped knit top. Her red curly hair is cut shorter, almost a buzz, and she sports a silver nose ring along with the stud in her eyebrow. "Hi, Heather," I say, touching her arm. "How are you today?" I cringe at the slick magazine. Tom has asked me to get rid of the "trashy reading material" in the waiting room but I've argued that women enjoy reading the articles. When else do we have time to catch up on Tom Cruise's love life or take quizzes on our sexual IQ?

"So how are things?" I ask Heather. The smell of the periodical's perfume advertisements fills the exam room.

"Pretty good, I guess."

Four words in a row. It's practically the most I've ever heard Heather say in her surprising soft alto voice. "Any bleeding or spotting?" I start charting her responses.

"No."

"Any cramps?"

"No."

"Have you thought about birth control?"

Heather doesn't answer, just turns a page. Then finally, "Do you think drugs could have made the twins die?"

"What?"

"Drugs? Can drugs kill babies if the father takes too much?"

I stop charting. Tilting my head to one side, I envision the thin, long-haired T.J. "You guys into a lot of drugs?" I ask casually.

"T.J. is. He was in the ICU last night. Overdosed . . . He's got IVs in both arms and an oxygen thing up his nose." Heather stares vacantly around the room. "I was there all night. They let me see him this morning, but mostly I was in the waiting room. I thought for sure he would die this time."

"It's happened before?"

Heather rolls her eyes and snorts, indicating this should go without saying.

"So what does he use? Heroin? Cocaine?"

Torrington is not the big city, but I've heard hard drugs are around. Some of my boys' old high school buddies have been busted, and I suspect they were selling more than grass.

The patient returns to the glossy magazine, contemplating an outfit that looks like it could be purchased at the Goodwill but is priced at six hundred dollars. Maybe Tom's right: we should get rid of these magazines.

"He uses some of everything," the young woman answers.

"And you?"

She shakes her head. "Not much, a little weed. What about the babies, though? Could his using drugs make them die?"

I have to be careful. I don't want to exaggerate or minimize. I don't want to create blame where there isn't any. "Well, it might be possible, but not likely. It's more dangerous if the mother takes drugs, of course."

"Can the drugs get in the guy's sperm and kill the babies that way?"

"No, I don't think so."

Heather nods thoughtfully. "Okay, I just wondered."

"So how *is* T.J.? You must be tired. Did you sleep at all?"

"He'll go to a regular room tonight. He might even get out to-morrow. I'm wiped out and I'm pissed at him too. I don't even care anymore. He can kill himself if he wants. It's not my problem."

I don't believe her. "Has T.J. ever tried to get counseling?"

"Nah. He says he doesn't need it. Says it's not a problem."

"Well, he almost died . . ."

Heather shrugs.

After the exam, I sit down again. "So we'd better get you on *some kind* of birth control. Even if you want to get pregnant later, it sounds like T.J. needs to get his head together. What do you think? Have you ever been on birth control pills?"

"I tried 'em before. I kept forgetting."

"Well, we have the birth control shot."

Heather shakes her head no. "I hate shots."

"Or the patch. The birth control patch is a method a lot of young women like. You don't have to remember to take something every day. You just put this small patch like a Band-Aid on your stomach once a week. I could give you samples, enough for two months."

"I guess." She doesn't sound enthusiastic.

I change the subject. "Heather, where is your real mom? Your grandma used to come with you, and she always seemed so mad."

Heather appears to study the advertisements for fur coats in *Vogue.* "She lives in Georgia."

"Have you always lived with your grandma?"

"Nah, just this year. I could have gone with my folks when they moved, but we fought all the time and then there was T.J. . . . . I used to think I loved him. So Grandma said I could stay, but then Gramps got sick and I got pregnant, so it hasn't worked out so good. I thought maybe T.J. and me would get married after the babies came, but . . ."

I see the tears and move closer.

Neither of us says anything for a moment.

"You think you'll be okay, Heather? I mean it. Are you going to be okay? I'm worried about you. You've got a lot to deal with, and a lot of women, most women really, after a miscarriage . . . well, you know, they feel kind of down. Even if they didn't mean to get pregnant, maybe they get excited for a while and then the baby's gone. It's hard." I remember my own three miscarriages, the sadness and anger.

"I'll be okay," Heather mumbles. She takes the samples of birth control patches I've laid out for her and then stands.

"You going back to the hospital to see T.J.?"

"Nah. He's gonna live. He can sort it out on his own. I can't carry his sorry ass around all the time."

I regard Heather. She needs hugging, but her emaciated shoulders warn me away. Then she surprises me. She leans over and gives *me* a hug. Her body is nothing but bones.

MRS. TERESI

Tom's pager has been going off all day in the clinic. In a lull between patients, I follow him into his office. "Everything okay?" I can see that it's not. His smooth face is blotchy and red.

"It's Dottie Teresi, my hysterectomy of yesterday. Her hematocrit is dropping, and she's spiked a temp. I think she may have a hematoma or an abscess but I can't get her a CT until late tonight. The nurses are freaking and calling me every few minutes. I'm going to transfer her to the ICU."

"Is she that critical? What's her temp now? Did you get blood cultures?"

"One hundred and three. Blood cultures are pending. Who do you think you are, the doctor?"

I shut up. I was only trying to be supportive, but we've been through this before. When Tom's hassled, he doesn't want my suggestions. I back into the hall. "Will you make it home for dinner?"

"I doubt it," he snaps. "I have to stay around the hospital until I figure out what's going on."

As I walk away, I realize that Tom's upset not just because Mrs. Teresi is ill but also because he's worried he may be responsible. The patient's husband, Dr. Teresi, a neurologist from Delmont, had personally requested that Tom do his wife's hysterectomy, and my husband had been honored. Now this happens.

Tom is one of the most skilled gyn surgeons in Torrington. He performs surgery on patients whom other physicians would refer out, women who've had multiple operations, women with adhesions and severe endometriosis, women who are malnourished or morbidly obese. Dottie Teresi had undergone three C-sections in her childbearing years and had a fibroid uterus. She'd been bleeding off and on for five months before she gave in and had surgery.

"It took me two hours to cut through the layers of scar tissue," Tom had told me at dinner last night. "The bowel and bladder were all stuck together; one of the most difficult hysterectomies I've done."

At 3:00 a.m. I'm still wide awake and wondering how Dottie is doing when my husband quietly opens the bedroom door. "Everything okay?" I ask. I watch him strip off his scrubs in the near dark, exhausted. He's been up for twenty hours and has to go back at six thirty.

"We gave her two units of blood. Her hemoglobin was five, now it's up to seven." I wince. This is still very low. "The CT shows that it's a hematoma, a collection of almost two thousand ccs of clotted blood. I'll try to have it drained by radiology in the morning."

Tom rolls on his side. I want to ask if Dottie is stable, if she's awake. I want to ask how Dr. Teresi is taking it. Is he upset and angry, or does he, being a physician himself, realize that these things happen, no matter how good the surgeon is? Tom's already asleep.

Raising up on my elbow, I stare at him in the moonlight. My husband has aged. It's the sag of the chin, the worry. Where before I hadn't seen lines, I see now that he's not twenty or thirty or even forty anymore, and his short speckled hair is more white than gray.

I look down at my lover, a man I've known since he was younger than our boys are now. The weight of his work is pulling him down. He doesn't say much, but he takes this so hard. Each financial problem, each complication, is another furrow etched in his face, yet inexplicably he sleeps like a baby.

"Hallelujah"

I open my eyes, and the light of the blue sun catcher is reflected on my arm, and "Hallelujah" by Leonard Cohen is still repeating on the CD player. I'm lying naked on the blue and white quilt with my husband curled around me. We're at the cottage on Pelee Island for a four-day weekend, a welcome rest after the worries about Mrs. Teresi.

This is the first time we've been away since June. It was hard to leave Torrington, and we almost didn't. His patient is still on a cooling mattress with a temp of 103. She has three IV antibiotics running, and the hematoma, which is now an abscess, is shrinking, but Tom worries her infection may be caused by a resistant strain of bacteria. Dr. Hazleton is covering while we're gone on this minivacation.

We'd made love after lunch. Now the sun's low in the sky, slanting golden across the lake and pouring in through the small window at the head of the bed. I lift up to look at Tom's face, so relaxed, so at peace. I haven't seen him looking like this in a long time, and I think of him as a young man and myself as a young woman, just starting our lives. I think of all the years we've been together and how much I still love him. Outside the open window, the waves of

Lake Erie lap at the rocks. Tom reaches out for me in his sleep, smiling, adjusting our bodies together. This man is a metronome for my days. He's what keeps our rhythm.

Sometimes life is too beautiful and too sad. The cells of our skin interlock like the notes in the song. *Hallelujah . . . Hallelujah . . .* I wipe my tears with one finger and gently wet Tom's cheek, but he doesn't open his eyes. "I'm getting up. I have to write."

Tom squeezes me tight and says, "Hmmmm," then lets me go.

There are only a few hours left before dark. I pull on my jeans and T-shirt, forget the bra. In two days we'll take the ferry home, go back to work, and meet woman after woman in the exam room. On the break wall, I sit on a granite boulder with my laptop resting on my knees. Writing the women's stories has become a compulsion. If I don't write them down, I'll forget.

I remember one story. It's Penny's story.

PENNY

"I like coming to you. I'd rather have a female doctor than a man. You're nice," says the thirty-seven-year-old when I return from the lab with her prescription and a handout about vaginitis.

"Thanks, that makes me feel good." I don't say anything about the reference to me as a doctor. I just let it pass. I've learned that patients feel bad when I correct them, as if they've somehow offended me. I wear a name tag that says PATSY HARMAN, NURSE-MIDWIFE-OB/GYN PRACTITIONER. They can read. That's good enough.

Penny Simmons is a thin, rough-looking blonde who's been, as they say, around the block a few times. Her pale skin is coated with pancake makeup, and she smells like cigarettes and perfume.

"I like helping patients take good care of themselves and making their exams as easy as I can," I respond and hand her the script for

Diflucan. "The microscope confirmed it's yeast. There was a lot of discharge. This medication should take care of it."

Penny takes the square piece of paper but doesn't stand up to get dressed and leave. "I don't like going to men. I had a bad experience with an exam once."

I'm at the sink washing my hands. I pull a paper towel out of the dispenser, taking my time. There's probably a way to ignore such a comment, but I don't know how to do it. "Was it a rough exam?"

"No, just the opposite. This was a long time ago, when I was seventeen. It happened at the family-planning clinic maybe twenty years ago. Family planning is at the health department now. Used to be at Torrington State University Medical Center." She waits to see if she should go on and takes her cue when I lower myself to the revolving stool.

"What happened?"

Penny stares down at her blue exam gown. "I went in for birth control pills. Me and Steve had just married and we didn't want to have babies too soon; just a birth control visit, but you had to get examined anyway." I nod. "He wasn't even a real doctor. He was a . . ." The patient searches for the right word.

"An intern? A resident?"

"Yeah, one of them. He was young. Didn't seem much older than me, but all dressed like a doctor in a long white coat. He kept saying he had to examine me. He made me come back three times before he would give me the pills. 'I need to check your ovaries. They feel enlarged' is what he told me. He would tear the paper exam gown open real slow. I didn't want to keep going to him, but the birth control pills were free and I had to get them."

I'm beginning to feel uncomfortable. This doesn't sound right.

Penny goes on as if she's merely the narrator of the story, not a participant in it. "So I came back like he told me. The last time he locked the door, and the exam took a while. I don't know how long. The whole thing was so embarrassing. I just stared at the ceiling.

He kept going in and out with his fingers. Touching me. I lay real still. Since I'd never been to a gynecologist before, or even talked to anyone about it, I didn't know what the exam was *supposed* to be like. I should have stopped him, but I was so shy. Now I would just kick him in the balls."

A resident in his long white coat. It had to be a resident, not a medical student. The students wear short coats. I picture it: He's standing between the girl's legs, stroking her, watching her face. Penny is pretty then, with long, naturally blond hair and pale skin. She doesn't try to get away. He smirks, convincing himself she likes it. Her legs are in the stirrups and he is standing so close. Now she's breathing hard. He's breathing hard.

I'm feeling sick.

Penny continues. "I don't know how long it lasted. Maybe ten minutes, but I had an orgasm." She slides her eyes over to see my reaction.

I'm speechless at first . . . then finally: "Did you ever report it?"

"Oh yeah, I was so upset I had to tell someone. I told my husband. He was only twenty, but he took me to the police. He said we had to *do* something, that the doctor should be arrested because it was rape. I hadn't thought of it like that. I'd felt it was *my* fault. So I went. It was awful. I had to tell the story over and over. More cops kept coming in and sitting with their little notebooks and writing things down. One cop told me it would be a hard case because it would be my word against the doc's. He asked me if I had gone to the emergency room to be examined for trauma so there would be proof, but there wasn't any trauma, so I hadn't gone.

"Steve had to wait downstairs. I don't know why, *just procedure,* they said. I could hear them laughing out in the hall. They took my statement and said they'd talk to the doctor, but nothing ever came of it. This was a long time ago. There were no women cops then. We were just kids to them, really."

For once I have nothing to say. I know unprofessional and exploitive things happen in health care, but a patient has never told me anything personal like this. So finally I ask, "Do you know who this physician is? Do you know his name?"

"No. I forget it, if I ever knew. I guess I wanted to forget."

"Did you ever get counseling?"

"I never confessed it to anyone else before. Not even Ma. She would have blamed *me*. Steve's been good, though. He talked me into getting my checkups again a few years ago."

"Did you ever see that doctor again?"

"I would never go back there. I imagine he's gone."

I want to know what the young doctor looked like, but I don't want to dredge up bad memories. Maybe the guy's still around somewhere, a pedophile stroking young girls, thinking they like it, thinking he's helping them develop their young sexuality, justifying it in his warped mind. I feel my face flush with anger. "Do you remember what he looked like?"

"Oh, I won't forget. He was tall, with thick hair; brown, I think. He had long fingers, thin fingers like a girl. Very handsome. I can't remember the color of his eyes. I don't think I really looked into them."

I take a long, shaky breath. I would like to hunt this pervert down, but I imagine he's long gone. Penny sits calmly, her head tilted, inspecting one of the framed photographs on the wall. It was a long time ago for her. To me, it just happened.

"This is like where I live," the woman says, nodding at the picture. "Where was it taken?"

"At the state park." The photograph is one of mine, a view of the forest in the fall when the leaves are in full color. There's a mist blurring everything, and the sun pouring through.

"I'm sorry all that happened to you," I say, apologizing on behalf of the 99.9 percent of doctors, physician's assistants, midwives, nurses, and nurse-practitioners in the world who are decent and caring people. Penny shrugs.

"Let me get you some samples of vitamins and calcium. Do you need anything else?" She shakes her head no. When I return with the bag, I want to hug the young Penny, the seventeen-year-old Penny. The middle-aged Penny is waiting near the door, her black cloth handbag over her shoulder, dressed in jeans and a bright red sweater.

❊   ❊   ❊

I close my laptop and look out at the golden sun setting into Lake Erie. I could have taken the photograph off the wall and given it to her. I wish that I had.

MRS. TERESI

My husband exhales in a drawn-out sigh. "What's up?" I ask.

"Huh?" We are hiking along the beach on Pelee Island, about a mile from the cottage. The waves lap up on a slate rock surface as smooth as poured concrete. A round boulder sits exposed, left by a glacier millions of years ago. The air smells of rotting fish.

"The long sigh, what were you thinking?"

Tom breathes out again slowly. "I'm just thinking about Dottie, Mrs. Teresi, and the phone call I made to the hospital yesterday. I was wondering how she is now, hoping she's better. When I called Dr. Hazleton from the Pelee Tavern, he said the clot was resolving and she was starting to eat, but if she gets febrile again I'll have to take her back to the OR for the third time. If the infection is resistant to the antibiotics, I'm not sure what I'll do." He pushes back his rimless glasses and smiles sheepishly. "I know," he says. "We said we wouldn't talk about work this weekend, but I'm still worried. Sometimes I think I just want to walk away from it all." He whistles for Roscoe, who's wandering along the edge of the lake but getting too far away. If that dog sees one rabbit, she'll run for miles.

"Remember when the phone rang at home the other night about three?" Tom goes on. "It was the nurses calling. I had this sense of dread that something else would go wrong and I'd be called in for a hearing in front of the peer-review committee." He picks up a stone and skips it across the water. "You know that happened to Dr. Runnion, don't you? Hal Runnion? He was harassed for two years by the committee. They're a board of docs authorized by the hospital to investigate surgical complications or medical errors, a real power group. They looked at every surgery Hal had ever performed, criticized him for every minor complication. Dr. Jamison told me he thought Runnion's competitors on the committee were trying to destroy him. If that's so, it worked.

"The peer-review committee has no checks or balances." Tom shrugs and walks on. "Their meetings are secret, the minutes protected by law. I don't know what went on in there, but he finally lost his privileges."

"Dr. Runnion? I remember it now. There was a big article on the front page of the *Torrington Tribune*. They made it sound like he was a quack, a danger to the community."

"Yeah, it ruined him, and the hospital's required to report any restriction of a physician's privileges to the National Practitioner Data Bank, on the Internet. After that, Dr. Runnion was finished, couldn't get liability insurance and couldn't get privileges anywhere else. He ended up having to close his practice and leave town. Too bad. He was a good doc . . . Really cared."

I listen, for once not saying a word. I've never heard Tom talk like this before.

"There's no way *any* surgeon can be without complications forever," he goes on, "especially with the cases I have. But when the phone rang, I thought, *I like my work and I think I take good care of my patients. I know I do. But this tension isn't worth it. I don't like being a surgeon that much.*"

"Do you think that's what's going to happen to you? Peer-review harassment? Like with Dr. Runnion? Burrows and Hazleton are on that committee, aren't they?"

My husband shrugs. We trudge on in silence, watching Roscoe run into the water and back.

Tom is a compassionate doctor, so careful in the OR, so competent, so calm. I know how much he's concerned about his patients, and the OR nurses like him. Many of them come to him for gyn care, and they're good judges of competence. It makes me sad to hear my husband ready to give up a career in medicine he's worked so hard for.

"We can quit any time," I say, reaching for his hand. "Maybe it would be for the best. There are lots of other things we love to do. Making ceramics, writing, photography, taking care of the honeybees." I pull him over to a smooth square boulder and we sit down. Far across the water, against the red sunset, two sailboats lean into the wind.

"Red sky at night, sailors delight. Red sky in morning, sailors take warning," I say aloud.

Tom stares straight ahead, not seeing any of it, not the silver water reflecting the pink and red clouds, the seagulls gliding across the bay, or the white sailboats on the horizon. "Unfortunately," he counters, "ceramics, photography, and honey don't pay the bills."

"But the boys will be out of college soon. That will help. We could put the house on the market, get a smaller place, and go back to being hippies. Well, sort of hippies . . . but we'd have to have indoor plumbing!"

I go on, pressing my point. "I could sell my photography. You could expand the beehives and market the honey." If we closed the practice, the worst part for me would be letting go of the staff, women who've stood by us since we started.

We rise and head back toward our cottage. Tom whistles again for Roscoe. She's as rebellious as our boys, and she runs the other way. Finally we catch her and put her back on her leash. The knot that had loosened in my stomach over the last few days begins to tighten again, like the collar around the dog's neck.

Later I ask him, "Do you think we should call the hospital and check on Mrs. Teresi after dinner?" We're at the Tim Goose Inn, the only gourmet restaurant on Pelee. It's our last night on the island.

"No, I'll call in the morning. Dr. Hazleton is competent to cover."

"But don't you want to *know* how she's *doing?*"

"No," Tom snaps. "I called yesterday. I don't want to hear about it until tomorrow, when we get back to Torrington. Even if she's worse, there's no way to get off the island tonight."

"It'll be okay," I say quietly, wanting to mean it.

"Yeah, probably."

Then we say nothing. After dinner, we pick up our bikes where we left them in the bushes and pedal back to the cottage. It's almost dark now. Roscoe follows on her leash as we roll through the dusk over gravel roads, past the campground with campfires burning and the marina with the little lights from the fishing boats. I think again how it would be to sleep without concerns about taxes, office finances, peer-review committees, surgical complications, or the suffering of patients. Tomorrow we will go home again, back to the cares of the world.

It has been a long time since the only responsibilities we had were to ourselves, our family, and God.

Dream of Flying

For three days I've managed without my sleep medicine. Tom's worried I'm drinking too much. Maybe I am, but I'm trying . . . I stand in the bedroom, listening resentfully to his soft snore, then open the glass door to the porch. High in the sky the crescent moon holds a bright star in its arms. I'm restless tonight and I don't know why;

I'm exhausted, but my brain won't turn off. With a shrug of disgust, I go back to the bathroom for the jam jar of scotch, then return to the deck chair overlooking Hope Lake.

Mica hasn't called for a month. If I say anything, he'll be consumed by guilt and even less likely to telephone. My oldest has a problem with guilt. I don't know if he got that trait from Stacy or me, but it wasn't learned from Tom. I don't think Tom ever feels guilty. We're out of milk and toilet paper. I should stop at the store after work. The thoughts free-fall through my mind as I stare into the woods.

It's quiet tonight. Then the wind comes up, and the alcohol settles me. "Thank you," I say out loud into the darkness. Thank you to whom? Thank you to God? Thanks to the booze? Thank you to the comfort of the dark forest and lake below?

At the foot of my bed I drop my terry robe and crawl in beside my gentle, hopeful husband. I sleep . . . then I dream:

Four women, naked under their thin blue cotton gowns, wait on four chairs in the exam room. They sit like a Greek chorus, muttering secrets they won't tell the midwife.

One is young and afraid. Her long brown hair hides her eyes. She's pregnant by her fifty-year-old stepfather. One is tall and impatient. Her coiffed wig hides her baldness. She has eight months to live. One is obese and ashamed. She has bruises on her back and doesn't please her husband anymore. One is shrunken and wise. She had sex with herself before breakfast.

From the corner of the exam room, I watch unseen. I too am naked under my exam gown.

Kneeling on the cold linoleum floor, I pray, adoring these women whose lives are as knotted and scarred as my own. The sun rises in the windowless exam room and the walls fall back.

Like a red hawk, I rise.

When I look back, the four women are flying with me, and their blue exam gowns open like wings.

*

Fall

CHAPTER 8

CAROLINE

The first day back in the clinic after a break is the hardest. It takes me a while to get in the swing.

This morning the office is tense. Donna is crying in the kitchen, but before I can find out what's going on, a petite Asian woman stops me in the hall. "Hi, Patsy. Do you remember me?" I've got other things on my mind, but I answer politely, "Mmmmm, you look *familiar*."

"You did my first delivery, don't you remember? I'm Caroline, the patient whose baby was breech at thirty-eight weeks, then head down, then breech again. Dr. Harman was planning to do a C-section, but just before going into the OR, he did one last scan and found the baby was head down again." She waits for me to remember.

"You're Caroline Akita." My face lights up. "How could I forget."

"I just wanted to say hi. I saw the other nurse-practitioner for my gyn annual. Your schedule was full."

As always, I'm apologetic. "Sorry." I give her a one-armed half-hug. Watching the tiny woman walk away, I think back to the birthing room. When was this, six months ago, a year?

❊   ❊   ❊

"So what do you want to do?" Dr. Harman is asking the patient after doing the final ultrasound in the triage room of the birthing center. "The baby's in position, head down again. You're already three centimeters. Maybe we should get labor started before the little guy turns again." We all agree.

Tom breaks Caroline's water bag with an amnihook, a slender plastic device that looks like a long white crochet needle. I write on the admission note, *Induction of labor at term, artificial rupture of membranes. Diagnosis: Unstable lie.* The fluid is clear, not bloody or stained, so Tom goes back to the office.

Two hours later, the patient is dilated to five centimeters. Contractions are coming every six minutes, but Caroline never groans, never moans, never asks for pain medicine. Once she says something in Japanese to her husband. The man places his hands on each side of her face and kisses both her eyes.

There's nothing much for me to do, so I observe from the rocking chair, occasionally murmuring words of encouragement. "You're doing so well." "That's perfect, Caroline." "Go with your body. Don't try to get away from the pain. The contractions will only hurt more."

Mozart plays on the boom box, the fetal heartbeat remains 145 with good accelerations, and the mother's vital signs are all normal: my favorite kind of labor. But when I do the next vaginal exam, I'm surprised to discover that the fetal head, which was engaged at zero station earlier, is now transverse and out of the pelvis, meaning that the baby has moved backward and is now turned sideways. This isn't good.

"How's she doing?" asks Jay, the concerned husband.

"Still five centimeters, but don't be discouraged. The baby's just trying to get into position. Time to get up and moving again, Caroline. Why don't you try squatting, and, Jay, you can stimulate her nipples. See if you can make the contractions stronger." The labor nurse, Joy, draws me toward the door.

"Everything okay?"

"The head's not engaged anymore. It's turned sideways now, transverse. I know I could start Pitocin, but Caroline's doing so well, and she wants to go naturally if she can . . . I'm going to give her two more hours, then if there's not good progress we'll augment her labor. You'd better check fetal heart tones more frequently, and I better level with the couple. Let them know what I'm thinking."

From two until four, Jay holds Caroline as she sways back and forth in a slow dance, one of his hands on her breast, twiddling her nipple. Contractions are now three minutes apart. When I next examine the young woman, I'm pleased to find the head back deep in the pelvis again and the cervix eight centimeters dilated.

"Why don't you start pushing, Caroline? Just lean on the baby, add a little oomph to the contractions."

An hour later, the patient is completely dilated. That's when everything hits the skids. As the baby begins to descend into the birth canal, the fetal heart rate drops below ninety. We roll Caroline on her side and I feel in the vagina for a thick rubbery cord coming in front of the baby's head, one of my worst nightmares, but there's no cord, just a little round head as hard as a potato. As Caroline's pain eases off, the fetal heart rate improves. Four more contractions, same story. Each time, the fetal heart rate falls lower, takes longer to return to where it is supposed to be.

"Call Dr. Harman, Joy. Tell him I need him here now." The nurse nods and bustles out of the room. I have dealt with many complications, including babies born with the cords around their necks, but part of being a good midwife is knowing when a patient might need a cesarean section and when to call an OB to your side.

"Oh *no*, I have to poop!" Caroline cries with big eyes. Then, realizing it's not poop, the young mother puts her chin to her chest and pulls back her legs, instinctively. Her labia open, and a baby's head, covered with black hair, is right there. The fetal heart drops again, this time to fifty.

"Push hard, Caroline. This is the most difficult part for the baby. Push like *your baby's life depends on it*."

The nurse returns, sees what's happening, and pulls up the

gooseneck lamp and the stainless-steel table. "Dr. Harman's on his way. It will take five minutes, maybe ten." She glances at the clock on the wall. Caroline growls deep in her throat, not waiting for Tom, and I don't want her to.

"Push!" I exhort. "Push like you mean it. Make every push count." I give a low, prolonged groan from deep in my abdomen to demonstrate. Jay, aware of the slow fetal heartbeat, bends low with his arms around his wife and grunts too.

Then suddenly the head is crowning. "Blow, blow!" I hold up my hand like a traffic cop. "I have to check for a cord around the neck and then you can push again one more time."

Running my fingers along the side of the baby's neck, I feel for a smooth rope-like piece of flesh. An umbilical cord around the neck is not unusual, but when I find this one and try to slip it over the infant's head, it's too tight. I try again, put some muscle into it, and this time the rubbery cable of flesh slides over. But wait! There's another loop.

"I got to push again!" yells Caroline as she uncontrollably bears down. "It's coming!"

"No! Blow! Jay, *make* her blow. There's more cord here and if she pushes it will tighten."

But there's no stopping Caroline now. As the baby emerges, his face dark blue from near strangulation by the umbilical noose, he lets out a cry and spins in my hands, unwrapping the cord that is still tangled around his chest and shoulders.

At that moment, Tom walks into the room, pulling a blue sterile gown over his shirt and tie. "Hey, nice work," he says, noting the crying baby I'm placing in Caroline's arms. "I shouldn't have hurried."

"Cord around the neck times two and twice more around the chest," I report, holding up the now flaccid rope of flesh, twice as long as normal. "It must be almost four feet. We've had deep decelerations with every contraction for the last fifteen minutes."

Tom pats me on the shoulder, understanding the pressure I was under.

"Nice work, everyone. No wonder your baby couldn't make up his mind which way to come out; he was dangling from a bungee cord." My husband smiles his wonderful smile.

❊   ❊   ❊

Such a special event, bringing new life into this world, how could I ever forget the Akitas' birth? Still, I comfort myself, there are so many birthing stories, more than a thousand, and even though I'd barely recognized Caroline's face, when she'd reminded me of the details of her delivery, it was all right there, her labor and birth, embroidered with colored thread on my heart.

"Better get a move on, babe. You're running behind." Celeste swats me on the butt with a yellow chart, and I drop with a thud back into the world of the clinic. Seven more patients to see before lunch.

At ten thirty, Dr. Harman shows up, wearing scrubs and two hours late for clinic. He doesn't speak to anyone, just grabs his stethoscope and heads for his first exam room. There's no chitchat among the nurses, no joking, no gossip, no stories about their families. When I get a chance, I pull Celeste into my office. "What's going on?" I ask her. "I saw Donna crying."

"It's her father. He had another heart attack and is over in the hospital. She didn't really want to be here but says working keeps her mind off what's going on with him."

"Shit."

"Yeah, it's bad . . ." Celeste lowers her voice. "What's up with Dr. Harman?"

"It's Mrs. Teresi. They took her back to the OR this morning. It's the third time. Her blood pressure was dropping and the general surgeon wanted to go back in. Tom won't even talk to me about it."

Celeste sighs, sweeps her dark hair away from her face, and clips it to the top of her head in an asymmetric ponytail. "I hate to see him this way."

"Are you doing okay?" I ask her.

She wrinkles her nose like something reeks. "Sometimes this place gets me down . . . the weight of it." A chime rings from Tom's exam room, signaling he needs a nurse. "Gotta go," Celeste says.

I press my lips together and stare out my office window. The leaves at the tops of the maple trees are just starting to turn red. Dark clouds in the west threaten rain. At least when I was in the birthing room with Caroline, there was nothing to worry about but one mother, one baby.

Yeah, I think, *sometimes this place gets* me *down too.*

TRISH

"Did you hear about Trish's daughter?" Donna whispers, pulling me aside as I enter the clinic, ten minutes late, on Wednesday morning.

"What?" I swing around.

"Aran's boyfriend, Jimmy, lost his job and ended up in intensive care after overdosing on Oxycontin." She bends in close, says conspiratorially, "Aran spent the whole night in the reception area *by herself,* waiting to see if he would pull through."

I lay my canvas briefcase down in the hall with more care than it deserves and go very still. "How did you hear that? Are you sure? Aran hasn't been seen in the office since she transferred to the teen OB clinic at the university, weeks ago."

"Vi, the receptionist in family medicine, told me. She heard about it when Trish called to tell them she'd be coming in late because she had to go to the hospital. Aran didn't even telephone her folks to let them know what was happening. Just sat up all night, *alone.*"

"Thanks for telling me, Donna. Is Trish in yet?"

"I'm not sure. Want me to call down there?"

"No, that's okay. I'll wait." All morning, women come in for annual exams, abnormal periods, and OB visits, but I'm thinking only of Trish and Aran.

By late afternoon Trish sits in my office, smoothing her daisy-print scrub jacket and crying. Her oval face is mottled and wet. "Well, Dan was right. Remember, he thought Jimmy was into drugs? But it's not just marijuana. It's needles and pills. He's out of the ICU and he'll survive, but he'll be hospitalized for another twenty-four hours. Of course, he feels terrible, apologizes for causing us trouble, tells us he loves Aran, and in his way I know he does. He promises he'll stop using, but he has no insurance and the bill will probably be fifteen thousand dollars." She wipes her nose with the back of her hand. I sit facing her, my knees touching hers. Trish pulls back her sandy hair with both small hands, staring out the window and watching her hopes for her pregnant daughter whirl away like the leaves off the autumn trees.

Finally I ask, "Where's Aran now?"

"She's sleeping. She called off work. Told them she was having contractions." Trish lets out a sad breath. "I don't know what to do anymore. Dan isn't speaking to anyone. He'd just like to lock Aran in her room. Keep her under house arrest. This craziness is tearing our family apart."

I gaze at my friend. I'm amazed that Trish manages not only to function but to do her job well in the midst of this chaos. She's such a steady, good person. "I don't know how you do it, Trish. What keeps you going? You feel like your family is falling apart, but you just keep on trucking."

My friend shrugs and raises one eyebrow. "What choice do I have? We're raising two other kids besides Aran, remember? They need some kind of life."

We stare at each other.

"Did I tell you when things were really out of control at our house, when the boys were getting into trouble, how I ran away from home?" I ask her.

Trish nods sadly. Yeah, she's heard the story.

Run Away

I share pretty much everything with my patients. I tell stories about myself. I tell stories about other women, about friends and patients. I'm always careful to change the place and time of the encounters because in a small community, you never know who knows who. I disguise the details, saying, "I had a patient once, this was quite a few years ago," or "This was when we lived in Ohio . . ."

Sometimes I tell mothers about the troubles Tom and I had when the boys were teenagers. I tell them how I wanted to run away. I was so tired of feeling afraid for them and feeling guilty that I'd screwed up. Sometimes I tell them that I did run away. This is the truth. It was around the time Orion was picked up downtown by the paramedics.

He was sixteen, I think, and was late for his twelve-o'clock curfew . . . the details blur after a while, fifteen or sixteen. Tom and I were in bed, but neither of us was sleeping.

The phone rang. Tom picked up. "Dr. Harman," he said in his doctor voice. The phone ringing that late didn't particularly alarm me. We were still doing deliveries and were often called in at night. What scared me was the way my husband sat up in bed and dropped his feet to the floor.

"When? . . . How are his vitals?" There were long gaps in the conversation. "I'll be right in." I felt nauseated. The word *his* was the tip-off. Our patients are female.

"What? What's happening?" I switched on the bedside lamp.

"It's Orion. The squad brought him into the university hospital's ER."

"An auto wreck?"

Tom pulled on his jeans. "No, he's in a coma." Our eyes met, saying everything. "Could be head trauma. Could be booze. His blood-alcohol level is real high. They found him in one of the row houses in the university student district. Someone called the squad, but no one was there when the paramedics arrived, so they don't know what happened. They're taking him in for a CT now."

"Should I come?" I started to get up.

"No, I'll call you." My husband left and I stayed in bed, praying.

When Tom returned, five hours later, he told me what'd happened. Someone had called the squad, but when the paramedics got to the Clifton Street address they found Orion abandoned on the floor of a trashed-out living room, hip-hop music blaring and a keg of beer on the kitchen counter.

Orion was in the hospital unconscious for seven hours before anyone knew whether it was an overdose or a head injury, maybe from a fall or an intentional blow to the head. It turned out to be alcohol poisoning. I think this was the same year Zen was expelled for having ten little baggies of marijuana on the high school campus after a basketball game.

During this time, I was insane with worry. The only one of the boys who seemed to be doing all right was Mica, in college in Connecticut. There'd been that incident when he'd worked as a pizza delivery man and was kidnapped by a group of thugs who'd forced him at knifepoint to drive to his ATM and take out money for them and then stole his car, but that was earlier. If he was in trouble now, we didn't know about it, and that was okay with me.

Those were the years when I began walking the floors. I stopped sleeping with Tom, camped in my study, and prayed on my knees, but I never missed work. I smiled and was nice to the patients. I told no one what was going on at home, that we were losing control of our children and that I was afraid if they didn't end up dead, they would end up in prison. I had no one to tell, no friends or colleagues who had kids being hauled in by the police or found almost dead by paramedics. The only thing that soothed me were my fantasies of flight.

Whenever I was alone, I would imagine a cozy home free of fear and fighting, some safe, calm haven. I would visualize myself packing the Civic, going into detail about what I would take: a few framed photographs, my favorite blue quilt, books, CDs. I pictured myself packing my guitar, my cameras, some kitchen things, a suitcase of clothes, a book of poetry. My escapist plans gave me peace, and I reviewed them over and over.

And then one day, something, I can't remember what, pushed me over the edge. It might have been Zen's acid trip when he thought he was God and we had to drive to Philadelphia to get him, or maybe it was when he stood in the TV room and called me a bitch. Whatever had happened, I went to the phone, found an apartment, wrote Tom a note, and left. I'd spent so much time thinking what I would pack, it was easy.

In the halls of the faculty OB clinic, Tom and I saw each other daily. We were professional and polite, but looked at each other with eyes like wounds in our faces. Sometimes Tom would visit my little furnished studio, which was as sweet and quiet and lovely as I'd imagined. There was a fold-down bed like in the old movies, a kitchenette, and a small dining table. I smoothed my patchwork quilt over the sofa and put up a few pictures on the white walls. Outside the front window I hung a bird feeder, and in the evenings, I would watch purple finches fight over millet and flax seeds.

"I want to move here too," Tom complained after we made love on the blue and white quilt. But we couldn't *both* run away at the same time. Someone had to be responsible and stay with the boys. I was gone for three months, and then one night after work I moved home and cooked dinner.

Now, when a patient confesses to me that her son is in jail or her daughter is out on the streets, I'll roll my stool closer and tell the mother my story. I tell it because there was a time when I told no one.

I told no one because I knew no one who I thought would understand.

NILA

"Hi, you didn't expect to see me back so soon, did you?" Nila looks about like she always looks: tidy, with her midlength blond-brown hair tied back in a ponytail. Her clear skin is now tanned from the summer sun. She wears size 2 jeans and a blue T-shirt that says WORLD'S BEST MOM on the front of it.

"I *am* surprised. So, how are you doing?" It's been months since Nila Wilson transferred to her new nurse-midwife, and I'd assumed she was settled in mid-pregnancy.

Follow-up gyn problem, the note on the chart says. Must be some mistake; Nila ought to be five or six, maybe seven months pregnant by now. I glance at the woman's belly, checking for the swelling that should be there.

The patient meets my eyes, placing both hands on her abdomen protectively. "Well, you probably heard. I lost it."

"No, I'm sorry, I didn't know. I guess the other ob-gyn practice didn't think to tell me . . . I'm really sorry." Nila begins to spill tears. I grab the box of tissues and slide my stool closer. "So what happened? How pregnant were you? Are you doing okay?"

"I lost it," Nila says again. That's all she says.

"But what *happened,* did you just start bleeding? What happened?"

"Yeah, I'm sure it's my fault. Doug told me to slow down. But you remember, I never had problems with my first seven pregnancies, and I kept working as hard as I could. We got that old place on Weimer Road. I told you about it, the big farmhouse? Well, it was a dump, but perfect for us, six bedrooms, two baths.

"No one had lived in it for years. The kids and I started with three rooms, the kitchen, the living room, and the one bathroom that worked. We got those livable and then we just camped out, cleaned and painted another room every few days. I mean *serious cleaning.* Some of the windows were broken, so there were leaves and bird nests everywhere, all kinds of shit." She checks to be sure her language has not offended, and when she sees that it hasn't, she goes on. "Literal *shit!* Bird poop, mice poop, some bigger stuff, maybe raccoon. It was hard work, but fun. The kids and I slaved all day and half into the night for two weeks. Of course, I was working harder than anyone through the heat of August. I was obsessed. Nesting instinct, I guess.

"All that time we were bringing in furniture, whatever we could scrounge or get at yard sales and flea markets. We got cheap paint at the discount place out on Bobtown Road and whitewashed everything. I couldn't ask Gibby for any of my old things, you know, my ex-husband, so we had to outfit the whole place. We worked our butts off, me and the kids. Doug was at Select-Tech ten hours a day, and I applied for food stamps.

"The first night Doug and I got settled into our new bedroom we made love. That's when the bleeding started. Doug blamed himself. I'd spotted once before, with my fourth pregnancy, so I told him it would be all right." Nila stops for a minute. I picture a stocky, good-looking guy in his early forties who hasn't had much to do with childbirth staring down at the streak of red blood on the sheets.

"But it wasn't all right. When I went to my midwife she couldn't find a heartbeat. They did an ultrasound, and the baby was dead. It wasn't the intercourse. I'm sure of it. It was all the hard work. I should have known better. I was four months along. I just thought I was superwoman. Now I know that I'm not. Eventually, I had to tell the kids. They didn't even know miscarriages happened, since all of my pregnancies had gone fine before."

Nila is quiet for a moment, remembering. She just sits there, a deflated balloon. "Then my sister, you know, Marnie?" I shake my head no. "Yeah, you do. She was at my last birth. Anyway, she's *real Christian* and she told me the miscarriage was punishment from God for adultery. You know how she is.

"If I was a drinking woman, I swear, I would have started right in. Doug was crying and blaming himself because the miscarriage happened right after intercourse. And Marnie was telling me it was some kind of holy curse, and the kids were looking all worried. I had to go into the hospital for a D and C. My doctor told us that miscarriages just happen sometimes, that it wasn't anyone's fault, but I don't know . . . *I was working too hard.*" Nila studies my face, waiting to see what I think.

"I agree with the OB," I tell her. "Sometimes the baby's not forming right, or the placenta comes loose. It hardly ever has anything to do with what you *did* or *didn't* do. One out of five pregnancies ends in miscarriage. Some say one out of two if you count the real early ones. You've just been lucky before. Will you and Doug try again? I know you were happy about the baby."

Nila shrugs her narrow shoulders. "Maybe, but I want to get the kids settled first, and then we'll see. School is just starting. And I want to get a divorce from Gibby. He's driving me nuts. When he heard about the miscarriage he sent me flowers, started calling, wanted to get together again. He says I wasn't meant to be with anyone else. He keeps going on that *our* babies always came out good, and I can't have one with another man . . . *I gotta get a divorce.* I'm thinking of going to some kind of legal aid. He's driving me nuts." She says it again.

I've never seen Nila so distressed. "Maybe I can help you with that. Didn't you tell me that Gibby had been hitting you after his head injury? Wasn't there something about that?"

"Not really hitting. He always stopped short."

"What, then?"

"Just picking on me. Telling me I was lazy, that the house wasn't clean, that I wasn't taking care of the kids. He'd get real angry but he never *hit* me. One time I thought he was about to. He shoved me against the stove and it was turned on. I burned my arm. He didn't mean it to happen, but I took the kids and went to Marnie's that night. A few weeks later, I left in the van." I remember Nila's impressive dawn getaway with the six kids.

"So did he *threaten* you with violence? Did he do anything else?"

"Oh sure, he *threatened*, but it was all hot air. He'd mouth off, say he'd kill me if I ever left. I didn't believe him. We'd been together forever. I know he loves me in his own way."

"Nila, I'm going to give you the number for the Rape and Domestic Violence Center. They may be able to assist you. There are lawyers in town who volunteer at the shelter to help abused women get a divorce."

Nila frowns. "I wouldn't want to get Gibby in trouble. I wouldn't want that. We were together for so many years and he's the kids' father."

I stop the discussion. I've heard this before. "Well, I'll give you the card with the phone number. At least you think about it. Gibby sounds potentially dangerous to me. If a man threatens you with death, it's serious."

"I'm okay now," Nila reassures me. "He sent me flowers, and I have Doug."

I smile resignedly. No use pursuing it, but I'll give her the card. We always keep a stack of them in the restrooms so women can take them without having to tell us their problems. "So what brings you here today? Have you had a period since the D and C?"

"Yeah, I'm fine. I just had a few days of spotting but I think I need to get some kind of birth control. I've never used any before. I read you shouldn't take contraceptives after the age of thirty-five if you smoke cigarettes, but I gave up the fags when I was in South Dakota. Could I get the birth control patch I've been reading about?"

"That's great. You quit? Not easy to do." I check Nila's blood pressure and write her a script for the patches. Then I give her a long hug. "I'm sorry about the baby," I say gently, patting the woman's flat stomach. Nila peers down at my hand. She takes my fingers and puts them up to her cheek.

"Thanks," she says. "Thanks for listening to me." There are tears in her eyes again.

Nila is scheduled to return in three months for a birth control check.

Superwoman.

HEATHER

"Hi, Heather, how're you doing?" I touch the slender young woman's shoulder as I enter the exam room. I'm mildly surprised to see T.J. standing in front of the mirror that's mounted on the wall in the corner, staring at himself. His long hair is gone and his head is now shaved. There's a tattoo of an eagle on the back of his neck, and two wooden plugs in his earlobes.

A few months ago, I'd written the patient a prescription for birth control patches; now her urine test is positive for pregnancy. "Hi, T.J.," I say, wishing he weren't here but obliged to include him. "Did you guys get a frost out your way this morning?" I have nothing against the boy, but the only time I've had any real communication with Heather was the time she came to the clinic alone. My conversational gambit flounders.

The kid shrugs. "I don't know. I wasn't up until noon."

Heather sits hunched on the end of the exam table in an exam gown that could wrap around her two times. Her arms are folded tightly over her front, and she's working her angular jaw back and forth. She glances up at me.

"So how *is* everything?" I begin. Heather rubs her bare feet together and shoots me a look. I notice her stubby nails are magenta now. Something is wrong, more strained than usual.

T.J. turns back to his reflection in the mirror. "New haircut?" I ask, to be friendly. *The guy's so self-centered* is what I am thinking, but maybe he just feels out of place.

He continues to inspect himself. "Nah, had it for a while."

"So what's happening, Heather? I see by the nurse's note that you're pregnant again. Is this something you wanted?" No eye contact. "Last time you were here, you were going to start the birth control patches. Did you change your mind or did you forget?"

"She didn't *forget*," T.J. mumbles.

"What did you say?"

"She didn't *forget!* She wanted to get pregnant."

"*You* did too!" Heather snarls. "You *said* you did, anyway."

I suck in a long breath. "It sounds like there's some tension about this." *That's putting it mildly.* I raise my inner eyebrows but keep my face deadpan.

"It's him," Heather says.

T.J.'s head snaps up and he glares at his lover.

"She already knows," the young woman continues. "I told her about the drugs."

I turn from my patient. "You still pretty heavily involved in drugs, T.J.?"

He rests his long, narrow body against the wall. "Some."

"What are you using?"

"Just grass, a little crack . . ."

"Any narcotics?"

T.J. glances at Heather, then at me, wondering how much I know. He fiddles with the thick silver wallet chain attached to his belt. "Not much, just now and then." I flip the chart back and forth, waiting.

"Just tell her, T.J. *You shoot up.*" Heather looks at me. "I *told* you. He shoots heroin and Oxy and any other thing he can get his hands on. I'm tired of it! I'm pregnant. I can't babysit him and take care of a kid too. Every night I have to watch him snort or shoot up, wondering if I'll have to call the emergency squad again. I'm fed up," she snaps at T.J. "For *real!*"

I sigh. I'm not in the mood to do couples' counseling, and the emotions in the room are swilling around me like sewage. "T.J., I'm going to assume you are a relatively intelligent person. It's not just that some of these drugs can eventually kill you, it's that the lifestyle that goes with them is incompatible with being a parent. You know what I mean? It's not an environment you want to raise a kid in."

T.J. gazes at the ceiling with disgust. "I'm going to quit when she has the baby."

"Right," says Heather.

"It's easier said than done, T.J. You may need some help. Have you ever tried a treatment center or therapy? I know some good drug counselors."

"I don't need help. It's not like I'm addicted. I've quit before."

"For about six days," says Heather.

"How about two weeks! Remember last year?" They're raising their voices.

I decide to change the subject. "Heather," I break in, "let me go over your OB dates and see how far along you are." I glance at the nurse's note in the chart and see that Heather has listed the bleeding after the twins as her last menstrual period. "No bleeding since the miscarriage?"

"No. Well, maybe one day, but just spotting."

"Did you use the birth control at all, Heather?"

"No." The girl is inspecting the bulletin board's colorful handouts on laser cosmetics and sleep problems.

Great. I look at the man, waiting for *his* excuse.

"You told me you *wanted* a baby," T.J. says, squinting at Heather.

Taking the round metal pregnancy wheel, I withdraw into my calculations and come up with her estimated date of delivery based on the last episode of bleeding, but it's just a guess. The young woman could have ovulated any time and may already be through the first trimester. I have the patient lie down on the exam table, cover her legs with the white sheet, and pull up the thin blue gown to her navel. "Any cramps this time?"

"None," Heather answers, staring up at the ceiling.

T.J. is squirming in his chair like a kid. I wonder why he even bothered to come but decide I should give him credit for trying to act like a man. When I feel Heather's lower abdomen, the uterus is easily palpable.

"I'm going to try to find the baby's heartbeat," I tell them as I place the small Doppler above the patient's pubic bone. "It's probably too early, so don't be disappointed if we don't hear it. I rarely pick it up before ten weeks." The room goes quiet, and T.J. turns to watch. At first there's just static, and then suddenly the faint click of the fetal heartbeat. I catch Heather's eye. Her gaze slips to T.J. He's alert, but unsure. "That's *it*," I exclaim, using my index finger to mimic the rhythm. Looking at the second hand on my watch, I count 140 beats per minute, a nice average rate for a fetus. "It's a good strong heartbeat. Congratulations!"

Both the young people are beaming now. "I think this baby is going to make it," I say. "There's never a guarantee, but I'm estimating that you're almost out of the danger zone for miscarriage." There are tears in Heather's blue eyes.

T.J. stands with his hand resting on his lover's narrow bare foot. Maybe there's hope for them yet. You never know what will make people change.

"So when do we get an ultrasound?" T.J. demands, slipping like a snake back into his old skin. "We need to know if there's one or two babies." He's standing too close. I can smell beer on his breath and I move backward toward the door. This guy's wound too tight.

"Since you're already nearly twelve weeks, Heather, and I don't think you're going to have a miscarriage, I'll be transferring you to your new provider next week. They'll want to do the ultrasound there. You'll need to get a medical card before your first visit at the new OB's office. I'm sending you to Sara, one of the other nurse-midwives. She's a little younger than me, but real nice. You'll like the whole group. There are three midwives and two ob-gyns."

T.J. is pissed about not getting the ultrasound and tries to act huffy, but he's not arguing and sits down. Heather has already started to dress, pulling on worn hot pink thong underpants and low-cut faded jeans.

"I'll get you some samples of prenatal vitamins." I stop with one hand at the door. "T.J., I want to say again that it's important, for you as a couple and for the baby, that you get this drug thing under control. This is no way to start a family. Will you try to get help?" The young man shifts his gray-blue eyes sideways then back. Finally, he nods without expression. That's all, one nod, and that's all I'm going to get.

A few minutes later, when I bring the samples of prenatal vitamins and the OB packet back to the exam room, Heather is tying her worn Adidas, and T.J. is already moving down the hall, anxious to leave. I watch his lean body turn the corner, power and grace like a ballet dancer. "Will you be okay with him?" I ask my patient. "I could try to find you somewhere else to live for a while."

Heather shrugs. "If he *tries* . . . I have to give him a chance, if he tries. He's the baby's father."

I've heard this a hundred times before. "He's the baby's father . . ."

Her young eyes look old.

Fear of Failure

With the two of us working, both professionals and one a surgeon, money shouldn't be a problem. It wouldn't be for most people, but for the last few years, our situation has been borderline and seems to be getting worse. Tom pays our household bills monthly, always writing checks for the minimum on our credit cards, holding the mortgage aside for a week if he has to. It's ironic. We're just like the average West Virginians, trying to scrape by, except we have more money, a nicer house, kids in private colleges, and bigger debts.

This morning Rebecca, our accountant, telephoned the office and asked Noelle, our billing secretary, if she had any checks to deposit. The quarterly installment for our medical-liability coverage, eighteen thousand dollars, is due at the end of the week, and we're four thousand short. Each year the cost of malpractice insurance goes higher, and Medicaid, Medicare, Blue Cross, and Aetna payments shrink. I wish Gorham wouldn't get the staff involved in our financial difficulties. They know we're not in great shape. When she calls like this and asks what insurance-reimbursement checks have come in, they worry about the practice's stability and wonder whether they'll have jobs next year, or even next month.

It's 1:35 a.m. I had just fallen asleep when Tom's pager went off. Now I'm up walking the floor in my white terry robe. Dottie Teresi has spiked a fever of 104, and Tom has gone back to the hospital. I don't ask questions anymore. "Good luck," I call out as he closes the door. For the first time it occurs to me that this patient may die. If she has an antibiotic-resistant infection she could slip into septicemia or go into cardiac arrest. I can't even remember how long she's been hospitalized. Though the general surgeons have taken over her care, Tom says he feels chained to her hospital bed.

It's become his whole lifestyle. He makes rounds on her at six in the morning, then sees her again at noon. He's back on her ward at seven in the evening, waiting to talk to her husband, Dr. Teresi. Sometimes, if she takes a turn for the worse, he goes in again later. Like tonight.

Unable to sleep, I decide to make myself a cup of Sleepytime tea. I'll try it, anyway. I swipe a cloth over the counter, staring around as the kettle heats. The dishwasher needs replacing. A white plastic panel came off the bottom six months ago and we haven't had the money or time to buy a new one.

Two years ago, when we'd hired Pete Burrows, we leased a larger office and furnished it; paid for his ads in the newspaper; invested in marketing; paid his salary, paid his malpractice premiums and retirement fund; and enlarged the staff. A big investment. Then we encouraged all new patients to see Pete while he built up his practice.

I take a sip of the tea and walk out onto the side porch. I still don't comprehend what clouded our judgment, or what we should have done differently. He *seemed* like a good man. We shared liberal political views, a love of nature, and a passion for the environment, but that wasn't enough.

Maybe we were just too hippie for him. Our ways of doing things and his ways were too different, and we couldn't talk about it. Pete resigned suddenly, taking his patients and leaving us with the costs of expansion. Later we realized he'd been planning his move for months.

It's like we were hit on the side of the head without warning, and we've never gotten back on our feet, never righted ourselves, never caught up. Pete still doesn't speak to us, and we don't know why. I shake my head, trying to lose the paranoia. How did a flower child who had faith that if you just trusted the decency in all people everything would work out become a middle-aged woman who can't sleep, she's so worried about everything? Reaching over the porch rail, I hold my hands open and let the starlight pour into them. I take the light and splash it up on my face. Four or five times, I let it pool and pour it over my head.

Then I take off my robe and walk down the steps into the grass, which is colder and wetter than I expected. With my hands raised, I dance in my short pajamas, dance in the moonlight at the edge of the garden.

I smell fall coming. You know that smell? The smell of dead leaves and rain. Then, with my hands clasped together, I kneel down in the wet grass and pray. Pray for Dottie Teresi.

REBBA

I am staring at a lavender envelope lying in the center of my desk, addressed in careful feminine handwriting to Patsy Harman. The return addressee is Rebba Tobin, Seattle, Washington. That name rings a bell. It must be a patient. Picking up the phone, I ask Noelle, our billing secretary, "Can you bring me Rebba Tobin's chart?" I spell the name out. "I *assume* she's a patient." Then I unseal the flap. Inside there's a flowered thank-you card, but the message is puzzling. No words, just a drawing. I frown at the cryptic symbols.

A few minutes later, Noelle steps into the office and hands me the yellow chart. Her normally composed oval face is flushed. "I'm sorry if I freaked out on you," she says sheepishly, shaking her head. "That woman in the waiting room was just really scary. I think she's an *addict,* and that boyfriend of hers, I bet she shares the pills Dr. Harman gives her with him. He gave me the creeps." She shivers and folds her arms over her chest.

Only an hour ago, I was standing in the reception area insisting a patient leave our office. I would have called Tom, but he was in the OR, so it was up to me. A stringy-haired, rail-thin redhead in jeans was pounding on the glass window, harassing the secretaries, demanding a script for Oxycontin.

"It's okay," I tell Noelle. "I was scared too, but not all patients on narcotics are alike. Remember that, okay? Most of them are fine and take their medicine the way Tom instructs them." Noelle shrugs and backs out the door. I can see she doesn't believe me.

Sometimes, we judge too harshly, I think. We've never walked in these women's shoes. As clinicians, it's difficult to know what to do. Pain is real. A health-care provider's role is to relieve suffering, but narcotics are addicting, and for the vulnerable patient, that's trouble. For others, narcotics make living bearable.

The angry woman this morning called me a controlling bitch and a few other unmentionables, but when she realized throwing a fit wasn't going to get her more Oxycontin, she finally stomped out the door. Afterward I was shaking and didn't know whether to laugh or to cry.

I take a sip of my Stress Relief tea, skimming Rebba Tobin's chart until I get to the last progress note. Now she comes back to me, and I smile. Rebba was the slim, auburn-haired girl, a flower in spring, who thought she was frigid. Months ago I'd given her detailed instructions on how to fix that. Apparently, my advice worked.

I glance through the window just as the sun shoots through the high cumulus clouds. Beams of golden light streak down like in the movies and I hear the chorus on high that goes with it.

Now the symbols inside the thank-you card make sense: a heart with a big smile and, underneath it, an oversize exclamation mark. At least *this* patient appreciates me.

The girl had an orgasm!

CHAPTER 9

Jeopardy

I can't decide if I want to vomit or go into the break room and eat three pieces of German chocolate cake. The name on the chart is Rae Blandon. It's a name that wouldn't mean anything if it weren't for the record's request clipped to the front.

I reread it carefully. *McKenzie, Rogers and Clager, PLLC, representing the family of Rae Blandon, requests all patient records be sent to them, including laboratory and radiology reports.* The signature on the request is not Rae's but *William* Blandon's, executor of the estate. He must be a son or husband. I don't know what *PLLC* means, but it's nothing good. And the signature of the executor can mean one of two things: Rae Blandon is mentally incapacitated, or she's dead.

McKenzie, Rogers and Clager. The names are familiar. I reach for the telephone directory and turn it over. These are the guys with the full-page color ad on the back of the phone book.

MCKENZIE, ROGERS AND CLAGER, ATTORNEYS AT LAW.
MEDICAL MALPRACTICE SPECIALISTS.
REPRESENTING INJURED PATIENTS AND THEIR FAMILIES.
IT'S ALL ABOUT GETTING WHAT'S FAIR.

In the center of the ad are three smiling men in black suits with red ties. *It's all about getting the money,* I think.

I study their faces and then turn back to the chart, trying to remember Rae Blandon, trying to remember her story. A tall, anxious middle-aged woman obsessed with her health? Was that her? There are so *many* anxious women. I flip back to the last progress note, two years ago. The patient had never returned.

My last exam is well documented. The patient was doing fine physically that day, but I'd made a notation: *Patient's sister dying of breast cancer after long struggle with chemo and radiation.* In Rae's history, I'd written that not only did Rae's older sister have breast cancer, her mother and aunt had it too.

When did she leave the practice? In the correspondence section I find a transfer form and a surgery report from the Torrington State University Medical Center. One year after her last visit, forty-seven-year-old Rae Blandon had received a double mastectomy for an advanced malignant mass with involvement of the lymph nodes. The report from the Breast Care Center had been filed in her chart, but I'd never seen it.

The previous mammogram twelve months before had been normal. I shake my head, puzzled. It wasn't like I could have done anything for the sick woman at the point we got the surgery report in the mail, except maybe call or send her a card. That would have been nice, but the chemotherapy and radiation had probably come too late. Was it my fault? Could I have missed something?

For the rest of the afternoon, between seeing patients, I meticulously study the records with the eyes of a malpractice lawyer. The woman had gone for a mammogram every year. Her breasts were dense and the radiologist had always qualified his report with the usual words that the mammogram was not infallible and should be used as only a *part* of the information when making clinical decisions. My notes indicate that there were no discrete lumps but that the breasts were fibrocystic. I'd even written, *Instructed patient in breast self exam.* Had Rae found the lump herself and gone directly to the Breast Care Center without calling me?

That night, still obsessed about the possibility of being sued, I leave the office early to avoid the five-o'clock traffic. I can't see that I was negligent. I'm sure I would have done a careful breast exam, especially knowing that Rae's sister was dying of breast cancer. But

I'm not perfect. It haunts me that as I did her exam, I could have been paying more attention to Rae's emotional pain than to her breast tissue under my fingers.

After dinner, sitting on the porch, I tell Tom about the request for records. It's the first time we've chatted in weeks. Dottie Teresi is now out of intensive care and improving. There's even talk of a discharge, though Tom's not holding his breath.

"Let it go," he says, holding my hand. "You do the best you can. You use your best judgment. You listen to the patients and you try to help them. It doesn't matter. You can still be sued. Most of these threats of lawsuits don't materialize anyway. Let it go."

I love my work, but do I love it enough to go though the fear of a medical-liability suit? I shake my head, squinting at the violet sky and the lake and the stars, trying to get some perspective on things. The full moon is just coming over the house, and there's the smell of drying leaves in the air.

The universe is endless, without a center and without an edge. Tom and Patsy Harman are just two little specks in the cosmos, two spirits trying to do some good on this planet.

I still feel like crying, and I'm not sure if it's because Rae Blandon is dead or because McKenzie, Rogers and Clager, PLLC, are getting ready to take me to court for ten million dollars.

ARAN

Aran goes into labor almost two weeks late, and the birth goes better than expected. My husband's required to take call one night a month for the department of OB-gyn at Torrington State University Medical Center in order to keep his surgical privileges there, so on rare occasions he's allowed to attend one of our own patients' births. Though the university hospital, not Tom, will get paid for the delivery, it doesn't matter. He promised Trish and Aran he'd be there.

"I was surprised to see Jimmy in the birthing room," Tom tells me as he crawls into bed at three in the morning. "He looked a little green." We laugh.

Tom's exhausted and hasn't shaved for two days, but he's relaxed and his eyes twinkle. I lie now in his arms, listening to the story by the light of the prayer candle, missing the smells of amniotic fluid and blood, the grunts and groans and ecstatic shouting of birth.

"Trish was with Aran as her labor coach," Tom goes on. "Dan stayed with their other kids in the waiting room. Aran squatted on the bed and pushed the baby out in twenty minutes."

"What did she have? A girl?"

"Yep, a seven-pound girl. Apgar scores nine and ten. She looks great."

Tom has to get up at six so I leave the detailed questions for Trish. How did Aran handle the pains? How long was she in labor before she started pushing? Did Jimmy help with the coaching? What did Dan think? We kiss a little, just enough to leave me lying wide awake; he's asleep before his eyes close.

The next day I go to the postpartum unit to help Aran breastfeed and find that she's already nursing. "I did it! *Almost natural!*" the girl says, smiling. "I stayed on my feet during labor just like you told me. I got in the shower the last two hours and they couldn't get me out. All I had was a little IV medicine at the end. I don't even have any stitches." She's wearing a new pink flowered nightgown and is still running on adrenaline.

Jimmy's there too. He's holding the seven-pound girl, tenderly wrapped from her toes to her chin in white flannel with a white knit cap on her head. I reach over and peek under the hat to look at her black curls and smell the new life.

Jimmy looks up, his brown eyes brimming with tears, his short red hair still plastered down over his forehead from sweat. "She's a rosebud of a baby," he says.

They name her Melody. Mellie for short.

PENNY

"You have a patient in room two." Abby, my nurse today, is dressed as usual in a gingham uniform, this time lavender checks. She stands in the door to my office and hands me a chart.

"You okay?" I ask. Now Abby's dad is in the hospital too. He had a stroke and is not doing well.

Abby shrugs. "I'm worried about my father, but it's my mom and my sister that are driving me nuts. They want me over at the hospital with them every minute, but I can't just leave work. I can't afford to take more time off." She sucks in a deep breath. There are tears in her eyes. "You know, my mom's losing her memory. She doesn't understand I have a job, I have family."

"First Donna's dad and now yours—"

"Yeah, I got to go." Abby flies off and I sit for a minute, giving my patient time to put on her thin cotton exam gown. All night the rain and wind sang together, and now, through the window, I see trees that only yesterday were alive with color are today half bare.

I flip the chart open and stare at the notations, not really reading. This morning I found a letter from the IRS in my stack of mail. I didn't want to open it, afraid of what I might find. We'd paid the twenty-one thousand dollars we'd owed them because of our former accountant's screwup. What now? It was a letter claiming we are behind in our last-quarter taxes. When I called Rebecca Gorham's office to inquire about what was going on, her receptionist had told me Rebecca was in Europe. The part-time secretary, a college student more interested in painting her nails than in accounting, assured me she'd have Mrs. Gorham contact us as soon as she gets back. I push back my chair with a giant groan then head heavily toward the exam room.

Tapping twice on the door, I slide in and ease myself onto the stool. "So how are you, Penny?"

The bleached blonde gives me a half smile. "Pretty good, I

guess." Her hair is showing dark roots and her nose is too big for her oval face, but she has pretty, full lips and round gray eyes. The problem's her skin. It's pockmarked and covered in thick pancake makeup.

"So what brings you here today? Do you just need a yearly exam or are you having some problems?" I press my aching back against the wall and wait. Penny sits at the end of the exam table with her arms crossed, the sheet pulled up to her chin. "Are you cold?" I ask.

"No, I'm okay." The patient's voice is low for a woman, the kind of voice you get with a sore throat or smoking. "I just need a Pap test and a refill on my birth control pills." Her eyes slip away.

I open the chart to review her history. The patient was in the clinic for vaginitis a few months ago. "Any further discomforts with yeast . . ." I ask—then I stop. What catches my eye is my last note: *Patient relates history of sexual seduction and abuse by gynecologist when she was seventeen.* Now I remember Penny, and I feel just as sick as I did before.

On automatic, I go though my usual health-related questions, thinking about the story the patient told me at her last visit. "It appears you've had a problem with your skin," I mention, just to get the image of the warped gynecologist out of my mind. "What treatments have you tried?" The scars on Penny's face are deep. Some are new.

The patient shrugs. "Over-the-counter stuff."

"Have you ever been to a dermatologist?"

The woman shakes her head no. "I just got health insurance this year."

I gesture for Penny to lie down. The patient complies but keeps the sheet pulled up over the exam gown. I listen to her heart and lungs. "Now I need to check your breasts." Penny presses her arms up tight to her sides. "Can you go like this?" I say, putting my hands up behind my head. Penny hesitates, and then follows my directions. The same sorts of divots I'd noticed on her face cover her arms.

"Penny," I say, taking her hand and inspecting her forearm carefully. "Do you have a drug problem?"

"No."

I scrutinize the other arm. "Then what's this, these marks?" Both arms are covered with the same fresh red and old white scars.

"I didn't know you'd be looking at my *body*. I thought this was a gyn checkup."

"Well, I'm concerned. How do you get these scars?" I ask again.

The woman stares at me defiantly. "I'm a picker. It's a habit. I pick." She spits out her words like bullets.

"You pick when you're nervous?" I glance at her face again.

"Yeah, I pick when I'm nervous, when I'm upset, when I'm stressed . . . I pick until I bleed." She explodes. I see Penny's pain then. "I've tried to stop, but I can't . . . I've done it since I was a teenager."

"What have you tried?" I run my hands over the patient's arms. "Have you gone to a counselor or a therapist?"

"A long time ago." Penny shrugs again. "It was a waste."

I have a sudden insight. "Did this start after you were abused by that doctor?"

"No, before that." She shakes her head, looking inward. "It was some before that."

I hesitate. "What started it? Do you know?"

Penny stares at me, then at the white-tiled ceiling. "My uncle."

"Your uncle? How long ago was this?"

The exam room is very quiet, no sounds from the hall. "What I told you before," the patient starts out, as if seeing it all on video. "My husband. He wasn't my first, or the gynecologist either . . ." I give up the exam and draw my stool closer. Penny continues, describing it like it happened in another life.

"I was thirteen. We lived in the country on Milford Pike. You know where that is?" I nod. "My mom worked and my uncle, her younger brother, roomed with us for a while. He was twenty-two."

I know the road. There's a nursery out there. The boys and I used to go out in the spring to buy plants.

"Did your uncle force you? Rape you?"

"Nah, not really." She stops. "Do I have to talk about this?"

"No, you don't, but you can if you want . . ." I picture the patient at thirteen. Her hair would be golden and long, her skin clear with maybe a few light freckles.

Penny hesitates, then begins. "At first I liked the attention and having a secret from my mom, who if you have to know is a hard-assed bitch." She looks away. "He told me he loved me . . . I had two younger brothers, but they played outside most of the time. That's when we'd do it. My dad was killed in the mines." I don't even blink. "My uncle, he told me if anyone found out, we'd both be locked up. I believed him."

"Twenty-two?" I ask. "Your uncle was almost a man, almost ten years older than you. Did that feel okay?"

Penny shrugs. I'm not sure if that means yes or no, but she goes on. "One day she came home early, my mom. She worked in the shirt factory at the edge of town and the power went out. You know the old shirt factory? It's closed now. She caught us on the floor of the pantry." Penny's face flushes and she checks from the corners of her eyes to see if I'm shocked. I am, but try not to show it. I'm picturing them on the uneven worn floorboards in the small corner room pumping away with their jeans half down when the mother comes in. *What the hell are you doing?* the woman would yell. *Get the hell off of her.*

"When my ma discovered us, we told her we were just goofing around, *that it was the first time and would never happen again,* but she knew the truth."

"So what happened to your uncle? Did he get in trouble?"

"Yeah, but it wasn't all his fault. My mom and grandparents got together and decided if he joined the army and didn't come back for twenty years they would forgive him and wouldn't involve the authorities. They didn't want trouble from the welfare department or the courts. My grandpa drove him to the recruiters in Pittsburgh the next day. I never even got to say good-bye, and I've never seen him again. It was a scandal, but they mostly kept it hush-hush from the rest of the community." She trails off. I don't even look at my watch.

"After that my mother never said my name again. She never forgave me; she turned bitter. I'd shamed the whole family. I wasn't allowed to go anywhere but school, not even with girls. That's when I started picking and had to go to a therapist."

My mouth is half open; I'm stunned, and I lay my head back on the wall. I have no clue where to go with this.

Penny shakes her foot nervously. I asked why she picked and she told me, but I'm unsure if the cause was the sexual relationship with her uncle or the subsequent rejection from her mother. "So, the picking . . . tell me about it."

"I just pick . . . I don't know. If I start, I can't stop."

"But doesn't it hurt?"

"Yeah, it hurts, but that's part of the pleasure. If I'm upset, it gives me something to do with my hands. The therapist told me years ago that picking is obsessive-compulsive."

"But you're ruining your skin. You're a pretty person." I stand up to start the internal exam. Neither of us speaks except for the simple directions I give, the words women have memorized at their gyn exams over the years. *Can you slide down? A bit farther. One more jump. That's good.* And, *Can you open your legs a little? A little more . . . I'm going to be touching you now.*

When I'm finished, I wash my hands, then lower myself onto the stool again. Penny sits up on the end of the table. There's a hole in the toe of her blue sock and she tries to hide it with her other foot. "What does your family say about the picking? Do they try to help you?"

"Well, my mom." Penny shrugs. "I don't see her. She's all but disowned me. But my husband tries. If he sees me picking he kisses me. He's real sweet, but then I just pick in secret."

I make a decision. "Would you like me to see if I can help? I have some ideas."

"I don't see what you can do. I won't go to a shrink."

"Well, that was *one* of my ideas, actually. I think it *would* help and I know a good counselor, but if you won't, you won't. I was also thinking about the microdermabrasion treatments we have here. Do you know about them?"

"I saw the handout and sign, but I can't afford it."

"That might not matter. I could give you free treatments now and then if you'd stop picking. I don't do this for everyone. In fact, I've never done it for *anyone* before."

Penny listens, touching her face, but then pulls her hand away and sits on it.

"The microderm machine sprays little crystals on your face. There's no chemicals. Then it sucks off layers of the dead skin. It will take off the scar tissue little by little. If I see that you're picking your face again, I'll have to give up the treatments. It won't be worth our time if you're making fresh marks."

Penny looks doubtful. "What about my arms?"

"I'd like you to stop picking them too, but I realize that might be asking too much at first. Just don't pick your face. Maybe we can help you with your arms later."

Penny frowns. "I don't know why you care. What's it to you if I pick?"

"I don't know . . ." All over West Virginia, all over Appalachia, there are women and girls with bad skin, rotten teeth, scars, and untreated deformities; what's this one woman matter?

"I don't know," I repeat. "I just *like* you. I want you to stop."

What I mean is *Because you've suffered; because you deserve something better.* But I leave it at that: "I just like you."

Dream of the Dance

All night I've felt sad for Penny, felt like sending her flowers. As if *that* would do any good, would give her back her mother, take away her pain.

"Breathe in . . . breathe out. Let your mind be at peace. Breathe in . . ." I peer at the clock. It's 3:00 a.m. My mind is clacking away like Donna's keyboard. I get up and slug down my sleep medicine. There's no sipping. Then I snuggle up to my husband, who didn't notice I was gone, and try once again. "Breathe in . . . breathe out." I try counting backward from one thousand and then I'm . . . I'm in an open meadow . . .

I hear music. It's a waltz, gentle and easy in the slanting green light. One-two-three, one-two-three . . . The melody is floating up from a golden dome. Curious, I run down the long grassy slope and open the door. The piano gets louder, the golden light brighter.

This is a ballroom, but there are only women here, women I know. Candles flicker from candelabra set into the walls. The music swells. There's Holly, wearing blue satin, dancing with Nora, who's dressed in rose silk. There's Shiana in green chiffon. Then Aran, Trish, and Nila move in.

A bleached blonde walks up to me. It's Penny, who picks until she bleeds. She holds out her arms, and we begin to waltz, awkward at first. One-two-three, one-two-three. I'm getting the hang of it now. Everyone's dancing, all the girls, all the women, in their beautiful rainbow dresses. Feet flash in golden slippers as we spin faster and faster, laughing, holding on to each other.

When Penny, my partner, throws back her head, all the scars on her face are gone.

Serpent

At 5:05 p.m. Linda sticks her curly red head in my office door. "I'm about to leave. There's a call on hold for you. Do you have a minute to talk to Blake Rogers, or should I take a message for tomorrow?"

"Sure, put him on."

She transfers the call, and I answer. "This is Patsy Harman, nurse-midwife, how can I help you?"

"Hi, Patsy," says a warm baritone. "Hey, thanks for taking my call. I know you're busy. I'm Blake Rogers; I represent the family of Mrs. Rae Blandon." Now I know the name, Blake Rogers of McKenzie, Rogers and Clager, PLLC. I go very still and my hand grips the phone.

"We've been examining some discrepancies in Mrs. Blandon's chart. There seems to be a few pages missing. I wonder if you could send us another copy? We could reimburse you."

Instant hot flash, but I don't say a word. I'd checked the copy of the records myself. Nothing was missing.

"Mrs. Harman?"

The snake. What was he up to? Why would he want another copy of Rae's gyn chart? Does he think he can catch us at something?

"Mrs. Harman?"

"Yes?" I say coldly.

"Would that be any trouble?"

"I'm not sure why you're calling me *personally,* Mr. Rogers. Don't you usually just send a written request? Is there something in particular you're interested in?"

"No, we just want to make sure we have a complete account of what went on with Mrs. Blandon."

I can't think what to say. How about *Are you going to sue me, you shit?* That comes to mind. I shouldn't be talking to this guy anyway. He isn't *my* lawyer. He doesn't have *my* interests at heart. I can feel my pulse pounding. Breathe in . . . breathe out.

"Well, you know, Mr. Rogers, I *am* awfully busy. Why don't you have your assistant return what we've sent and I'll have someone go through the chart to see if anything's missing. I rather doubt it. As I remember, Rae was not a patient here for very long."

There's a pause on the line. "Very well, if that's the way you want things." The voice has gone reptilian. "We'll get that request in the mail tomorrow." He hangs up.

When I finally stop shaking, I grab my coat and leave the empty office running. Driving up the hill into Blue Rock Estates, I'm gripping the steering wheel so hard I can't swerve in time and crunch a baby rabbit under the right front tire and I start to cry again. When I open the front door, Roscoe tries to squeeze out and I hear that I've left the stereo on.

I miss Tom. What optimistic thing will he now say about the serpent Blake Roger's call? Tom's cup is perpetually half full. Mine is half empty, not even that. Sometimes I think that without him, I would spin into darkness.

Stripping off my tailored slacks and striped blue shirt, I notice a streak of red in my underpants. It's the second time this month I've had bleeding. I'd thought I was through with all that. It must be the stress. Then I flop on the bed in my sweats. A Grateful Dead song fills the room. How many times has it played today?

We will survive, the song says. *Things are bad and getting worse, but we will survive.* The music is infectious, and I smile in spite of myself.

I take a deep breath. "Yeah? No matter what? *We will survive?*" Outside, the last of the sunset shows blood red over the mountains under dark clouds.

If I weren't so wiped out, I'd get up and dance. I lie there on my back and dance with my arms. I can't help it. It's that kind of tune. *We will survive. We will get by.*

The song says so.

CHAPTER 10

Falling Stars

It's a clear evening with the bare black branches silhouetted against a lavender sky. I sit waiting at the window with my Stress Relief tea. Tom and I were going to go riding, but he had a call from Dr. Leonard Noble, medical staff director and chairman of the peer-review committee at Community Hospital. All day, Tom's been tense, worrying that Dottie Teresi's case will be brought up and some kind of restrictions will be put on his privileges. Leonard Noble is a legend in the Torrington medical community. The former thoracic surgeon, who has Parkinson's disease, is now the hospital's chief of staff. I met him once and have never forgotten his intimidating, narrow dark eyes, the way he has of looking right through you. I don't trust him, and I'm worried about Tom.

The front door opens, and Roscoe runs wiggling to her master. I hear Tom's briefcase hit the tile floor. "In here," I say. "How'd it go? Want some tea?"

"Yeah. I gotta use the john first." I go to the kitchen and pour another mug from the still steaming red kettle. I'm biting my tongue, trying not to ask everything at once, as I usually do.

Tom comes up behind me loosening his tie and hugs me.

"So . . . ? How was it?"

"Not so bad. We didn't talk about Teresi at all."

"No? What was it, then? What was the meeting for?"

"It turned out it was about that new guy who's interviewing for the CEO position. Noble wanted my perspective."

"That's all?"

"That's pretty much it. I was the one that brought up clinical issues."

"Like what?"

"I told him I planned to work with another surgeon as my assistant instead of an OR tech from now on. Most of the group practices already do. It will make it harder to get patients scheduled for surgery if I have to ask Dr. Hazleton or Parsons, but it's better to do it voluntarily than to have limits put on my surgery. And I'm not going to take medical students or residents from the university into the Community Hospital OR with me anymore either. I was really worried after Dottie's long hospitalization. The hospital lost money on that one. Want some wine?"

"Sure," I say, giving up on the tea. I've been trying not to drink alcohol other than my sleep medicine except on special occasions, but I guess this qualifies.

After dinner, sitting close on the porch in our pajamas and robes with a thick down quilt over us, we finish the bottle of chardonnay. It's a clear dark night, no moon yet. I slip my hand between Tom's legs under the cover. He's staring straight down into the woods at the reflection of the lights across the cove. "What are you thinking?" I ask.

"Oh, just how much I like the quiet. You know. Just fantasizing about what it would be like not to have to worry about this stuff, just imagining another life." He grins.

I'm feeling a little light-headed and move my hand up his thigh. Not much reaction. I fool around a little. "Remember, I suggested before that we could quit. I'm still willing. Maybe you could get a job teaching anatomy at the medical school."

Tom raises his eyebrows. "Spend all day in the lab cutting up cadavers with the smell of formaldehyde?"

"Well, there wouldn't be any complications! No peer-review committee watching over your shoulder. No lawyers ready to sue you!" This cracks me up.

Tom smirks at me sideways into the dark. "Right." He finally notices my hand. "Let's not talk about work now, okay?"

We kiss in the dark. He's been so low lately. I've been looking forward to doing something nice for him. It turns me on. Laughing, we spread the quilt on the porch floor and throw the other half over us, squirming around to get comfortable.

Then I hold on while we soar through the night. Afterward, lying on our backs, looking up, we see three falling stars.

HEATHER

I'm sitting at my desk reading, with relief, a long overdue e-mail from our accountant, Rebecca. *I returned from France last week,* she says, *but now have the flu. Don't be concerned about the quarterly taxes. I applied for an extension before I left. There's nothing to worry about. I'll work on them next week.*

When I look up, I find Linda from the front desk standing at my office door. "Yesssss?" I draw this out in a comical way like the evil boss on a TV sitcom. I'm in a good mood.

"Did you see my note?" she asks, not clowning around. There's something stiff about the way she stands there.

"What note?" I turn back to my keyboard. I'm finishing my reply to the accountant, asking for a meeting to discuss the practice's finances. My desk is a mess, covered with unopened mail and little yellow stickies to remind me of all I should do.

"I left you a note this morning. It's about Heather Moffett. I was looking at a week-old *Torrington Tribune* and there's an article in the obituaries. I think it's Heather's boyfriend."

Linda leans across me in her pink gingham-checked scrubs, her red ringlets falling, and rummages around on my desk. "Here." She pokes a piece of white paper at me. The sheet has an obituary neatly cut out and taped to it. A question mark is scrawled on the side and

Heather Moffett printed on top. I carefully read the short notice. *Thomas Joseph Morris, nineteen, died at Torrington State University Medical Center. He is survived by . . .* It was ten lines.

"Shit!" I shake my head. "I just can't believe it. First Heather loses the twins and now this . . . And she's still pregnant with his new baby. Have you guys heard anything?" Linda and Donna grew up in Torrington and are acquainted with or related to half the people in town.

"Nope, not really. I knew he was into drugs though. Big time. It was probably an overdose. The paper doesn't say, but I bet it was an overdose. I'll get you the chart."

"Yeah, I'll have to call Heather." *Shit.*

After lunch I find Linda has clipped Heather's phone number to the young woman's yellow chart and placed it in the middle of my desk. I try five times to reach her but can't. There's a fast beeping sound, like the phone's off the hook. Later my receptionist leaves a different number and note on my desk: *Call Heather Moffett.* I notice there's an unfamiliar area code, and I remember that the girl's parents live out of state.

This time it's answered on the first ring. A woman's crisp voice. "Moffett residence."

"Yes. Hi. This is Patsy Harman in Torrington. Is Heather Moffett there?"

"You are . . . ?" Said suspiciously.

"Patsy Harman, nurse-midwife, in Torrington, West Virginia. I used to be Heather Moffett's OB provider, her midwife. I was given this number to reach her." I'm cleaning up my desk with the phone tucked under my ear.

The woman's voice brightens as she recognizes the name. "Oh yes, one moment please . . . *Heather!*" she calls.

An extension's picked up in another part of the house and a soft, low female voice comes on cautiously. "Hello?"

"Hi, Heather. It's Patsy, Patsy Harman at the women's clinic in Torrington. How are you doing?"

"Oh, hi." Even lower, giving up all pretense of cheerfulness.

"I heard what happened to T.J. I'm sorry . . ."

"Yeah, T.J. is dead."

Heather's voice is so faint, I have to strain to hear it. My hands grow still and my heart very quiet. "I just read about it this week. Linda found the notice in the newspaper. I've been trying to get hold of you but there was no answer at your old place. Where are you, anyway?"

"I'm with my folks in Georgia."

"Are you okay? I mean, I know you aren't *okay*. But are you hanging in there? How's the pregnancy going?"

"Fine, I guess. Everything's fine *that* way."

"And the baby is growing? Kicking and everything?"

"Yeah, it's good. It's moving a lot." There's still no enthusiasm. "I just feel so *bad*. It's *his* baby and he'll never get to see it." There are tears in her voice, and for a moment the silence hangs on the phone lines. "T.J. overdosed. I never even got to say good-bye." You can tell that she's crying. They say it's therapeutic to cry but sometimes there's a limit to how many tears you can shed.

"You told me you were afraid something would happen to him." I picture the lean, graceful T.J. "He'd been in the hospital before."

"I *knew* it would happen. When I left Torrington, I just *knew*, but I couldn't stay with him. I was working my butt off, remember? I worked at the Discount Supply Depot, the warehouse down on the river. I liked my job, but I was six months pregnant and sometimes I was so tired I would almost faint. He told me he couldn't get work, so I was supporting us. No matter how tired or sick I was, I showed up. We needed the money.

"Then I found out he *had* a job. Can you believe it? All this time he was working, spending his money on drugs, and I was busting my butt to pay rent." She takes a breath. "I found his pay stub one day, and I let him have it.

"Well, that was the last time I saw him . . . He stormed out, slammed the door. I just sat there and cried." She pauses to blow her nose and clear her throat. "I was working so *hard* and all that time he had a cake job, getting ten dollars an hour at an auto-body shop and spending his money, money we needed, *on dope.* I never even got to say good-bye—"

Someone from a distance says, "Heather?"

"I'm all right, Mom." Then the girl's voice breaks again. "I blame myself. I *knew* it would happen, but I just couldn't stay. With a baby coming, I just couldn't live with him anymore." There's another silence.

"Oh, Heather," I say, cradling the phone as if I held her, "I know you feel guilty. Anyone would. But it wasn't your fault. You know that. You *have* to forgive yourself."

We talk some more. "I have a good doctor," Heather tells me. "He's the same one that delivered me. I just feel so sad that T.J. will never see his baby. I think it will look like him. It's a boy, by the ultrasound . . . I just feel so sad."

I take a deep breath and let it hang.

Celeste comes into the office quietly and sets the timer on my desk for three minutes, alerting me that a patient is ready in exam room 2. She pats my shoulder, noticing my tears and knowing by the chart open on my desk to whom I'm talking.

"Well, I gotta go. They have a patient waiting." I wipe my eyes. "Heather?"

"Yeah."

I want to tell her that the pure light within her will guide her way on, but instead I say, "Will you call me when the baby comes? Or anytime. Tell the nurses I said you can interrupt me if I'm seeing patients. It's okay." We say good-bye and there's no way I can hug the young woman.

On the way home from work in the Civic I sing the song I learned on the commune. I sing it to Heather: *May the long time sun shine upon you, All love surround you, And the pure light within you, Guide your way on.*

Circle

I have my women's meditation group at five and end up leaving a pile of charts stacked in the corner of my desk again. I've attended this group every other Monday for more than a year and it means a lot to me. Until we stopped delivering babies, I didn't have time to make friends. Now I sit in silence for twenty minutes every other week with women my age who wear Birkenstocks and jeans or long skirts and sandals. Half of us grew up in West Virginia. The rest moved here when we were hippies. Two of the women remember visiting our communal farm near Spencer, but that was twenty years ago. Zari and Carolyn have a homeschool consulting business, and Jean is a therapist with her husband. Mandy is a technical writer and Alice an artist. Three of us are nurses of one kind or another. Two are retired social workers. Almost everyone but me works part-time.

After our meditation we discuss books on Buddhism or radical Christianity. We eat bran muffins and carrots, or maybe a fancy souf-flé or scones, if someone feels creative. And *chocolate.* Can't have a meeting without chocolate!

Today I keep thinking about motherhood. When you have children, you unlock yourself to pain. Not just the contractions of child-birth, which split a woman open like a seed, but the pain that will inevitably come later, the pain of a son's broken arm or his broken heart. The pain of his loneliness, rejection, or failure. Sometimes the pain of his death.

I shift in my seat, flashing on Heather, all the hurt and grief she's had in her young life already, losing the twins and now T.J., all the pain she still will go through. I shut my eyes tight and pray a strong prayer, directing the energy from this group of women toward her. And toward T.J. too. May he find peace.

Then I focus my attention and follow my breath. Breathe in again slowly. The universe breathes too. The tide rises and falls. An acorn sprouts, grows to an oak, then dies and nourishes another kernel of life. The puddles of yesterday's rain evaporate and come down again as a cloudburst. I pray for my sons, that the stars will dance with them, that the sun will befriend them, that the radiance of the full moon will enfold them . . . Breathe in and breathe out . . .

The women are stirring. "Let us come back to the room," Zari says.

At the end of the meeting we hold hands, then bow to each other like Buddhist monks, with our palms pressed together in front of our chests. I am so honored to be with these women, all of whom glow.

"*Namaste,*" we say, looking into each other's eyes.

"I greet the light within you."

HOLLY

"You know these medications are habit-forming, don't you?"

Holly Knight slouches in the guest chair, stretching her long legs out across the exam room. She has puffy dark circles under her eyes and looks like hell. I continue my lecture. "Not physically addicting, but habit-forming. If you use them too much you won't be able to go to sleep without them, not even nap." I don't tell Holly how I know this. I don't tell her about the forty-eight sleepless hours I went through downstairs in our guest room one weekend to get them out of my system. I don't tell her about the sleep medicine in the little jam jar I use now.

It's a quarter to twelve, and a drug rep is serving us luncheon in the conference room today. I don't care about the food, but it's bad form not to show. We like getting their samples of birth control pills, hormone replacements, and antidepressants for our patients. We accept their lasagna, tossed salad, and cheesecake in return for a five-minute lecture on why their products are better than others.

"So except for sleep problems, you doing okay?" I soften. "How are the hot flashes?" The patient's not herself today, seems distracted and frazzled, and I decide to slow my inner clock and pay attention. "Are the hot flashes worse?"

Holly shrugs. Her usually coiffed hair is pulled back in a low ponytail; she wears no makeup. I've never seen Holly without makeup. Her face is blotchy and lined, making her green eyes look bigger, like they're swallowing her face, and there's a yellow pallor just under the skin. "Are you doing *okay?*"

I glance at her vital signs on the chart. Blood pressure and weight look good, pulse is fine, everything's stable. "So what's going on? Is it menopause, what?"

"It's the night sweats. They're happening again. And the mood swings. I'm losing it . . . I'm not sure if it's hormones or stress." I wait, let her tell it. "Nora's in the ICU again. It's the same old thing. I knew when she started spitting up blood that I had to do something. John says she has to *choose* to stop being bulimic, that she has to choose to live. But she has to be in her right mind to choose, doesn't she?" I nod. I've never seen Holly like this before. She pulls her hair back from her face, adjusts the ponytail holder, and wipes her tears with the back of her hand.

"It was awful last week. Nora was beside herself. She would run in and out of the house screaming, 'It's *my life!* I can do what I want with it.' I couldn't calm her down. Nothing seemed to work." Holly stares at her clenched fists. "We never did anything to hurt her, always helped her. Sometimes I'm so angry. This hurts me so much . . . but I know she hurts more. I just don't understand it. John says it's out of our control now."

Holly shakes her head. "She has to *want* to live. I know he's right, but a few nights ago, after I thought she was sleeping, I went to her bedroom, just to check, and there was blood all over the pillow. She was hemorrhaging. They think it's her esophagus. She looked so white in the dark, for a minute I thought she was dead. Then I saw she was breathing, and eventually she opened her eyes. I was on my knees and her breath smelled so bad. Old blood was all over her teeth. I took her face in my hands and I whispered, "We have to go. I have to take you to the hospital. *I can't let you die like this.* I wanted to shake her."

I can see it. Holly is crying. Nora is crying. *All right, Mom, I'll go. I'll go if you want me to.* Then the long-limbed mother crawls on the bed and holds her leggy daughter. Holds her like a baby, and rocks her too. The girl is so weak from starving herself and raging against the world that she doesn't resist. Outside the bedroom window the first flakes of snow fall in the dark.

Holly continues. "I didn't beg her to eat like I usually do. I just cleaned the blood off her face with a warm cloth and took her to the hospital. They're giving her hyperalimentation, electrolytes, protein, and fluids by IV. They think they'll be able to save her. They have to." She stops. "I just don't know what we did to make her this way."

I take out my pad and write scripts for the sleep medication and a slight increase in Holly's hormone therapy. She's waiting for me to say something, but I don't know what to say.

I reflect to myself that *we are not such screwups,* she and I. Holly was just an ordinary mom doing what she thought was right. We both love our children. Did we give our children too much? Did we give them too little? The exam room fills with our collective guilt and mother love. We are drowning in it. Finally I struggle to the surface.

"Okay, John might be right," I tell her. "Nora has to want to live. She has to want to live and get well. But it's in your nature to try to save her. That's what a mother is programmed to do. It's what we have to do, if we can."

*

Winter

CHAPTER 11

PATSY

"You bleeding?" Tom asks as we get ready for bed a few days after Thanksgiving. He stares at my pink cotton underpants in the laundry basket.

"Off and on. Not that much. It's just spotting. It doesn't happen every month."

"Why didn't you say something?" He's brushing his teeth and the foam dribbles out as he talks. "We should do an ultrasound and an endometrial biopsy. You know being on unopposed estrogen can cause endometrial hyperplasia."

"It's probably just a period. I'm cramping a little." I reach around him for my hairbrush. "My periods used to be irregular. It hasn't been that long since I stopped." I'm thinking it's no big deal. "Did you call Rebecca Gorham today?"

Tom shakes his head, no, but he's not diverted. "You're on estrogen replacement without progesterone, you have to get regular ultrasounds. Tomorrow get an appointment with me, and I'll do one. We should have done it months ago. And no, I forgot to call Rebecca. Why don't you talk to her? You have more time." He's crabby tonight. He pulls back the quilt and adjusts his pillows.

"I already left two messages. She hasn't returned my calls. She better not be in Europe again. If you telephone her, it might have more clout." I jump out of bed to blow out the prayer candle, placing my hand on the round wooden box. "Peace be with you," I whisper. Orion, Zen, Mica, Heather, Aran, Trish, Holly, Nora . . . everyone.

"Will you *please* help me out and do it tomorrow?" I ask again. "We haven't had a meeting with her in months."

Tom mumbles something and then he's asleep. As usual lately, I lie there resenting him. I'm weary of worrying about the practice problems while he sees patients and sleeps like a babe. I remember Mrs. Teresi and take back my malicious thoughts. The man works his butt off, what can I say. I'll try to call the accountant again myself in the morning and be more insistent with her little cat of a receptionist.

My ultrasound doesn't happen the next day or the next week, and neither does the meeting with Rebecca. I'm busy seeing patients and getting ready for Christmas, and then I stop spotting.

Most women do fine on a combination of estrogen and progesterone. I'm one of the exceptions. The progesterone makes me so depressed I can't stand it. When I finally have Donna pull my gyn chart, I'm surprised to see that my last ultrasound was ten months ago.

Now it's six in the evening, already dark, and Tom and I are the last ones in the clinic. I lean on the open door to his office. "Hey, want to do an ultrasound on me tonight?" I ask, as if inviting him out on a date.

He turns slowly from his computer. "Tonight? You still spotting?" His white shirt is rumpled and his tie is pulled loose.

"I wasn't, but it started again. Really, it completely stopped so it just slipped my mind."

Tom throws down his pen. "*Give me a break, Patsy.* You're really being irresponsible here. You've got to take care of yourself. We talked about it, what, a week, two weeks ago?" I feel like a schoolgirl reprimanded by her favorite teacher. He's right and I know it. "Okay, come on." He stalks past me.

We go back to the exam room. I've already turned on the ultrasound machine and typed in my name. I skip the blue exam gown and sheet, just pull off my slacks. Tom puts on gloves and gently inserts the vaginal transducer.

"Ovaries are fine," Tom says. "The endometrial thickness is excessive, though . . . way over."

I can see that he's right by looking at the monitor screen. My pear-shaped uterus is lined with white. "How much?"

"Fifteen millimeters. It should be under five." This is not good. "So, a biopsy?"

"Yep. Should have had one months ago." He shakes his head. Tom's not pissed anymore, just worried. He carefully inserts a small pipelle the size of an IV tube into the opening of my cervix and withdraws bloody tissue to be sent to the lab. It hurts, but I do my childbirth breathing and it's over in minutes.

"So I guess I better get started on the progesterone, huh? Make myself have a period and get rid of that stuff?"

"I'd say so," says Tom. "But I don't want to be your doctor on this."

"You don't want to be my doctor?" I'm shocked and a little hurt.

"No, this is potentially serious. You need to see someone else. I can't take care of you. If you need something done, I can't do it."

"Like what? Like surgery?" I frown. "It won't come to that. I'll start the progesterone tonight. I know I should have been doing it all along, at least every few months, but it makes me so low."

In the lab I dig around for some samples of medication. I'll have to take the pills for almost two weeks. A few days after I stop the progesterone, I'll have an artificial period, which will get rid of the excessive bloody tissue. Meanwhile, we'll wait for the results of the sampling Tom did tonight.

Unopposed estrogen can cause uterine cancer, but I've had biopsies before. They were fine. This will be fine too. Sometimes Tom Harman gets on my nerves. In the bathroom I swallow two progesterone pills. *Might as well get the show on the road,* I think grimly, looking at my face in the mirror. When I check my pink cotton underpants, there's more blood.

ICY

I'm stuck in a line of vehicles on Turkey Run, a narrow blacktop that runs between the agricultural school and the freeway. It's five o'clock, as close as you get to a rush hour in Torrington, and I'm on my way home from work, listening to a CD of John Sousa marches. I'd be better off on days like this if I rode my bike, only there's no berm to ride it on. To my left, the sun is dipping behind the bare trees. The stirring music reminds me of Icy, a patient I saw in clinic today.

Icy Miller is an eighty-six-year-old widow, a fluffy, soft, pink-skinned, white-haired lady who lives at Valley Manor, a retirement village not far from the office. I was the first woman she'd ever seen for a gyn exam. Now she sees me four times a year for a pessary check and cleaning. The three-inch rubber device, shaped like a doughnut, is worn by some older women in the vagina to support a vaginal prolapse. It's an alternative to surgery. Icy's in good health except for her blood pressure. At eighty-six, she still drives her own car.

In the exam room I ask Icy how she is. "I'm fine really, just having a problem."

"What's going on? Didn't I see you just last month?"

"Well, it's a little embarrassing. I went down to Florida to see my sister and I got real constipated. I strained too much and now the pessary's out of place."

"Did you fix your constipation?"

"Oh yes, days ago. You know how it is when you travel. You don't take care of your bowels, you don't eat the foods you're used to."

I help Icy lie down and put her narrow arthritic feet in the footrests and then with a gloved finger carefully remove the pessary. It was halfway out and rubbing the side of her vagina. Simple for me. Not so easy for her.

"So how's the rest of your health? Did you have a good time in

Florida?" I stand and wash the rubber disk at the sink, looking over my shoulder, taking my time. It's a treat to hang out with Icy. There are some patients you just like, you don't even know them that well and you like them. It's their life force or something. I replace the pessary with a little push.

I'm finishing up, writing a few notes in the chart about the short visit. "Do you know where you'll get your flu shot this year, Icy? There may be a scarcity again."

"No, I don't. I went to Dr. Sutton last week, he's my internist, and they don't have them, don't think they can get them either. I don't know what this country's coming to that we can't make our own flu shots. We seem to have plenty of money to throw around the Middle East." Her brown eyes snap in her wrinkled pink face and I raise my eyebrows. *This is interesting.*

"You think that's a waste?" The patient turns sideways on the exam table as easily as if she were a girl, and leans forward. "Of course, and I think it's *wrong.* What do they think they're doing with our American boys and girls? Throwing their lives away. It makes me sick, really. This country is falling apart, the economy and all. And that money we're spending over there, it's over *three hundred billion dollars* already and it will be over *five hundred billion* before we get out! Maybe a trillion. Think of the highways and hospitals we could build. Think of the schools and housing for the poor."

Right now, I look out my side window at Turkey Run Road, full of potholes, the berm washed away. I had no idea; could Icy be right? I think of the homeless; the high school dropouts; the loss of lives in the war, ours and theirs; the amputees . . . five hundred billion dollars?

"You know what, Icy? I think like you do, but I rarely say so to patients. Dr. Harman and I used to go to marches and sit-ins. Now we donate money to a few causes, but otherwise I don't say much."

"Well, you *should.* Not enough people say what they believe. That's how the government gets away with it."

I wince, knowing she's right. "But don't you suppose it would offend my patients?"

The line of vehicles on Turkey Run moves ten feet forward and I'm now only two cars from the intersection.

"Oh, honey, you won't. They know you love them and take good care of them. You might even have a good influence. That's one of the privileges of getting older. You get to say what you believe. Your words are worth something. You need to march on."

"You think so?"

"I know so!" The patient's brown eyes sparkle. "Now give me a hug."

Mrs. Miller throws out her arms and I move into them against her big soft breasts. She smells like cedar, good sense, and courage.

It's finally my turn to cross Bobtown Road. I wait for two minutes and at last shoot through the traffic. Then I open my window, turn up "Stars and Stripes Forever," and let it blast, not caring who hears or who it disturbs.

PATSY

It's been a brilliant blue day, cold and clear, and the sunset is just as radiant. Tom and I have finished dinner, stir-fried vegetables with chicken. We sit now in the living room, watching the sky turn from gold to red to lavender, until it's dark. As I rise to carry the dishes into the kitchen, he clears his throat. "The pathologist called about your endometrial biopsy today."

"And . . . ?"

"It's complex hyperplasia with atypia. He can't rule out endometrial cancer."

"I don't get it." I understand it isn't good, but I don't know how bad.

"Well, it means you have an overgrowth of abnormal cells in your uterus that could be cancer, he's not sure."

"What's he think?"

"Pathologists don't *think*. They don't guess. That's why they say 'a low-grade carcinoma cannot be excluded.'" My husband pulls the printed biopsy report, which is neatly folded in quarters, from his front shirt pocket. I spread it out on the kitchen counter and read the words twice, then go back to rinsing the stainless-steel sink. I feel Tom watching, but I don't look up. I've just been pushed off a cliff and am falling.

"I didn't want to tell you at the office."

I'm having a hard time hearing. The wind is roaring too loud as I plunge, tumbling over and over again.

"So what do we have to do to find out?" I say finally, shaking my head to clear it.

"Well, the usual treatment is a hysterectomy."

I'm sick with remorse. If I'd gotten the ultrasounds on a regular basis or told Tom when I first started spotting, this might not have happened. I'm always so busy, in so much of a hurry. Now I may have cancer, and it's my own fault.

"So what are the chances?" I ask as we return to the living room. The Christmas tree, decorated with tiny white lights, birds of all kinds and golden pinecones, sits in front of the windows that face the lake. The smell of Scotch pine fills the room. "I don't feel tired or ill. I don't think I have cancer. Shouldn't I have pain or be losing weight? I feel great."

Tom shrugs. "The thing is, I can't take care of you in this. I told you. I can't be your doctor."

"*I know that,*" I snap. "I'll find my own doctor. I just wondered, if I were your patient sitting in your exam room, what advice would you give me?"

"Have a hysterectomy. Then the problem is solved. You can use estrogen and never worry about taking progesterone again *and* you'll know you don't have endometrial cancer because you won't have a uterus." He smiles a half smile, thinking that's amusing, and squeezes my hand.

I don't squeeze back. "I told you, I *really* don't want a hysterectomy. Aren't there alternatives? It just seems wrong to have a hysterectomy if we don't even know *for sure* I have cancer." It pisses me off. I know that the removal of a woman's reproductive organs is the second most common surgery performed in the United States. Cesarean section is first. Each year, more than six hundred thousand are done. One in three women in the United States has had a hysterectomy by age sixty.

Tom shakes his head and lets his air out. "Okay," he says. "We can do a lit review on the Internet. I'll get on PubMed. What do you need to know?"

"Well, I want to know what the chances are with this kind of endometrial biopsy. What's the chance I have cancer? Fifty percent? Five percent?"

"Yeah, endometrial cancer grows slowly so we have some time."

"No, I need to know tonight."

Tom shakes his head and reaches for me. "Come here." I scoot across the couch, and he wraps his arms around me. "It will be okay. Even if you have a hysterectomy, what's the big deal?"

I draw back to stare at him. He doesn't get it. Jumping up, I move to the Christmas tree. "I just got over surgery with the gallbladder eight months ago. I hated it. I felt so vulnerable and out of control. It was one of the worst things that have happened to me."

"You did fine. You recovered great once you got home."

The smell of the pine needles fills the room as I stand with my back to him, randomly crushing them. "And what about sex?" I ask, wiping my tears surreptitiously. "Don't you care about that? Sex won't be the same."

"Actually, that's not true. They've studied that," Tom says this in his doctor voice. "The majority of women after hysterectomy have more frequent intercourse and more pleasure." He sounds like an actor in a white coat playing a physician in a TV ad. "More frequent intercourse and more pleasure—"

"Yeah, right! That's because most of them had pain before the surgery or were bleeding all the time, so of course sex is better. I see those women in the clinic, the same as you. Some even have worse pain *after* surgery because of adhesions or scar tissue at the top of the vagina."

The room is illuminated only by the miniature Christmas lights. I pace behind the couch and love seat, crying again, but he can't see.

"It won't be the same! When I have an orgasm I use my whole body. I feel the contractions in my uterus as much as my vagina. How would you like to have an orgasm without a penis?" I'm getting carried away here. Tom slides down on the sofa, looking up at the ceiling.

"Well?" I ask.

"Sex is ninety percent in the mind."

"So you don't think a woman needs a uterus?" I'm offended and irrational but I can't stop.

He stands up. "Let's cool off. We don't have to do anything tonight. Do you want an appointment with Dr. Parsons, Dr. Hazleton, or Terrance at State?"

"I don't care," I say, pouting. "How about Dr. Burrows?" This is a joke and Tom knows it. "Okay, Eleanor Parsons, I guess. I'd probably be more comfortable talking to a woman about sex . . . if it comes to a hysterectomy."

For the rest of the evening we research the incidence of uterine cancer with a biopsy result of complex hyperplasia with atypia. We peck away on our computers, each in our separate studies. I'm surprised to read that the chances of my having cancer are 30 percent. More than I thought. I still don't think it's that likely.

At midnight we go to bed. We're lying back to back and Tom reaches around and gives me a pat.

"Don't you worry about sex, Tom?" I ask softly into the dark.

"Not too much. I think you'll be fine. I know you better than you know yourself." He adjusts his pillow. "You'll be fine." In a few minutes I hear his breathing slow down and know he's asleep. *Mr. Positive.*

Tom always anticipates the best, while I am full of doubt. I could turn to hold him, to let him hold me, but I don't.

I completely forget to light the prayer candle.

❖   ❖   ❖

At the end of the week, Tom and I have an appointment late in the afternoon with Dr. Eleanor Parsons, a gyn surgeon in Delmont. The waiting room is a 1950s sort of space. Signs all over the glass at the receptionist's desk remind patients they must pay at the time of service, and blue vinyl chairs without armrests are lined up facing a TV mounted high on the wall. A lone secretary glances at her watch as she greets us with a clipboard of forms.

"Mrs. Harman," she calls a few minutes later and opens the door to the inner office. She is apparently both receptionist and nurse, and we follow her down the narrow hall, past the empty exam rooms.

At the door to her office a sturdy woman with sandy gray hair stands waiting. "Well, come on in!" the physician shouts, sounding as if we'd just come for a party. Eleanor Parsons is wearing a flowing black jacket with a leopard-print top over black narrow slacks and is holding out her arms. I tower over her. After giving us both big hugs, she graciously indicates we should take the two leather chairs across from her cherrywood desk. Her private office makes up in elegance what the waiting room lacks.

Before leaving the university and starting out on his own, Tom had worked with Eleanor on the ob-gyn faculty at State. For a few minutes, the two physicians chat about their children and what it's like to be in private practice, and then Dr. Parsons turns to me. Tom had called ahead, so she knows the story.

"So how are you feeling?" she asks in a soft South Carolina accent. I've been inspecting her paintings on the wall, the huge desk, the bookcase, but I rejoin the party; after all, it's for me.

"Okay, I guess. We've been thinking about what's the next step, and we've done some research."

"Well, I did some research last night too, after we talked." She's looking at Tom. "It isn't standard of care, but since Patsy can't take progesterone orally, I agree, the progesterone IUD may be the way to go. It will control the thickness of the endometrium without having a systemic effect."

I'm relieved that *hysterectomy* wasn't the first thing out of Eleanor's mouth. The two surgeons go on to discuss the protocol. Dr. Parsons's face is lined and pale, but there's a great kindness in her. She turns to me. "So when would you want to get the D and C, Patsy?"

"Soon. As soon as possible after my period."

"Assuming there's no cancer and you get the progesterone IUD, we'll have to do close surveillance if you want to stay on estrogen," Dr. Parsons continues. "This will mean frequent ultrasounds and possibly endometrial biopsies, and I'll be in charge of making sure the ultrasounds and biopsies get done." I know she's aware of my recent negligence, and I nod in agreement.

We stand to leave, pulling on our winter jackets, and Eleanor gives us each another big hug. I'm in good hands.

✻   ✻   ✻

For the next week I continue to take the progesterone with only a few serious meltdowns. I work eight hours a day, catalogue-shop for the boys' Christmas presents, fill a shopping cart with something for everyone at the bookstore, and breeze through the holiday sales at the mall.

At work, I go through the motions of caring for patients without caring very much about them. I ask briefly about their menstruation, bowel and bladder habits, diet and exercise. I take medical histories. I perform their gyn exams. I don't ask about stress, sleep problems, sex, or depression. If a woman's anxious, exhausted, or sad, I pretend not to notice. This is how providers who keep to their schedules must manage.

The staff all know about the abnormal endometrial biopsy. "Why don't you just have a hysterectomy and get it over with?" Abby asks me.

"*I* would in a minute," joins in Celeste. I know they're being supportive but I don't want to explain, don't want to tell them about my fears of not being able to have an orgasm. That's something I wouldn't even mention to the women in my meditation group. Yet I talk to women in the exam room intimately about sex every day.

On the ninth night, I gulp down the last two tablets of progesterone just to get it over with. That makes the ten doses. Then I settle down to wait for the withdrawal bleed. I still haven't said anything to our boys about what's going on. It will probably turn out to be nothing.

※　※　※

Two nights later, I begin to bleed. By bedtime, I'm changing my pad every two hours, and in the morning I check into same-day surgery and Dr. Parsons scrapes and sucks what's left of my endometrial lining out of my uterus and sends a sample of the tissue to pathology. I work the next few days as if nothing has happened. I haven't even told Trish what's going on; maybe she's heard. I just don't feel like discussing the shame of my negligence, how I've screwed up my body.

Tom checks twice daily on his computer for the pathology report. We don't talk about the future. I don't think about it either. I'm sure that I don't have cancer.

※　※　※

For the past three years, we've had our office holiday luncheon at the Riverview Inn on the Friday before we close the office for Christmas. At home after the party, I ask Tom, as I take up my knitting, "By the way, did you check the computer for the results of the D and C?"

"Yeah, it's back."

"It is? When was it posted?"

"This morning."

"Why didn't you say anything?" I reach over to untangle the blue yarn attached to the scarf I've just started for Mica.

Tom stands at the end of the sofa, still dressed in black Dockers, white shirt, and his holiday tie with holly and berries. "I didn't want to ruin the Christmas party."

"You've known all day? You could have told me."

"I didn't want to ruin the party," he says again.

I still don't get it. "So, what did it say? The pathology report?"

"It's cancer."

There may have been more but I didn't hear it. The echo shuts everything out.

C A N C E R . . . CANCER . . . C a n c e r . . . cancer . . .

I knit four rows. "That's all it says, 'cancer'?"

"No, it said, 'Well-differentiated adenocarcinoma.'"

I knit another three rows.

"So there's no choice," I say finally.

"No." He flops down beside me. He doesn't reach out, and I don't either. The shiny silver knitting needles flash in the candlelight. I want to run away, but there's nowhere to go. I'd just take the cancer with me.

"So when can I have the surgery?" There's no quibbling now. You want to live, you have a hysterectomy.

"Tomorrow," he says.

I nod.

Cancer! The word is still rolling around in my head like a boulder after a landslide. No one in my family has ever had cancer.

"Don't we have patients in the morning?"

"The staff will cancel them. I've already called Dr. Parsons. We're scheduled for seven in the morning. Everything's set."

Before bed, I e-mail the kids, the women in my meditation group, and a few friends around the country and ask them to hold me in their thoughts. In between e-mails, I knit twenty-three more rows.

After lights-out, Tom and I lie under the covers, holding hands. It's the first time we've touched since he told me. "Don't you care about sex?" I ask quietly.

He reaches for me but doesn't say anything.

"Do you want to make love?" I continue. "This is the last time I'll have all my parts."

"Sure," he says, chuckling, tilting my face up to his. He has the softest lips, full and tender. I run my hands down his belly and then lower.

In the end he climaxes . . . I want to but can't.

Still holding me, he says, "Don't you need to cry?"

I want to but can't.

❊   ❊   ❊

Early the next morning, I check into the surgical center with my knitting and my insurance card. That's one of the perks of being a gynecologist's wife. You need gyn surgery, no problem, you're on the schedule the next day.

Nurses I met last time when I had the gangrenous gallbladder, and more recently the D & C, nod, but no one stops to talk and no one meets my eyes. I think they know why I'm here and are distancing themselves. Then again, maybe they're busy. Tom plans to continue seeing patients at the office until they take me back to the OR, then he'll assist Dr. Parsons with the hysterectomy.

Silently, a medical assistant escorts me to a cubicle in a large pre-op bay with fifteen or twenty beds arranged around the perimeter and I'm told to get into my thin cotton gown and put my clothes in a plastic bag. Only flimsy peach curtains separate the spaces where men and women wait on wheeled cots for their IVs and pre-op lab tests. I can see their shadows on either side of my cubicle. They have family with them, and I listen to their low conversations while I undress.

I can tell by their dialects how different the families are. One group is from the mountains, maybe farmers, the other from the academic community, but they're each trying in their own way to distract their loved ones. The patients, me included, are all the same under these blue cotton gowns. Naked and scared.

I part the curtain so the nurses will know that I'm ready and get out my knitting. The soft blue yarn is a comfort. Even though Mica lives in Atlanta and will have little use for a wool scarf, I want to finish before Christmas.

Then an RN wearing a poofy paper surgical cap and reminding me of Nurse Ratched in *One Flew Over the Cuckoo's Nest* comes by with a clipboard and takes my vitals. She pumps up the blood pressure cuff like it's a flat tire, but I don't complain. Next there's the anesthesiologist, and finally Dr. Parsons.

"How you doin', hon?" she asks, sitting on the edge of the bed in her green scrubs. "Nervous?"

"I don't know . . . I'm shut down right now. Just going for the ride and wanting to get it over with."

"Well, try not to worry. I really think things will be okay. I do. I just have a good feeling."

No one has said the word *cancer*.

❧   ❧   ❧

I'm sitting in the living room a few days later, wearing loose knit black pants and a red sweater and looking like nothing has happened, when the boys begin to arrive for the holidays. First Zen with Callie. His shoulder-length straight brown hair is now cut in a buzz. He throws his blue parka on the floor and opens his arms to me.

"So, how you doin', Ma? You look pretty good." Zen is jolly, Callie quiet and concerned. Young women like Callie have come in and out of my boys' love lives for years, and I would adopt them all, but I've learned to guard myself, see how long they'll last.

Around midnight, Orion arrives with his hound. It's snowing, and he's driven six hours from Cincinnati after leaving his job at the art gallery. He parks his backpack and leather jacket neatly in the hallway and knocks on our bedroom door. Dozia, his unruly dog, comes in and jumps up on the bed, and I grab the pillow to protect my incision. "Hi, Mom. Hi, Dad," he says softly into the dark. "Down, Doze!" He pulls at the animal's collar. "I just wanted to tell you I made it. The roads were a bitch." He leans over the bed and gives us both hugs, pauses a beat, then retreats to the refrigerator. "Love you," he whispers as he closes the door.

The next morning Tom picks up Mica and Emma at the Pittsburgh airport. They come in about noon, stomping snow. Mica's shirt collar is half up and half down, sticking out of his trench coat, and I resist my impulse to straighten it. Emma's long fawn-colored hair wisps around her thin face. They make a good pair, both rumpled and elegant, brilliant and organizationally challenged. Unlike Zen and Orion, who have brought handmade gifts or intend to shop at the mall last-minute, Mica is laden with presents, all stylishly wrapped in green and gold holiday paper by a paid professional. I am careful to be cheerful.

The Christmas tree has been decorated for weeks. I'd put up a wreath and the manger scene when I first accepted that I might have surgery. This is minimal. I usually go all out. In the next few days, I do my best to participate in family activities, but mostly I sleep, recover from the surgery, and wait for the final pathology report that will tell us how far the malignancy has spread.

"If the cancer has gone more than fifty percent through your uterus, you'll need radiation," my husband tells me. But with all the festivities, there's no time to discuss what that means.

"How many days will it take until they post the report?" I hear Mica asking Tom in the kitchen.

"Sometimes as long as a week. With the holidays, maybe longer." Nobody speculates. Nobody discusses the odds, and the house is in continual commotion. The boys' old friends from high school arrive to visit. There's wrapping paper, ribbon, and Scotch tape everywhere. Shoes and boots pile up by the front door. Wet coats and hats are draped over the banister.

Ordinarily it would bother me, and I'd be buzzing around trying to organize everything, but it doesn't matter to me this week. In the midst of the chaos, I'm alone in a clean white waiting room with rows of empty white wooden chairs. I sit in the silent room, staring at nothing, just waiting to find out how far inside me the black cancer has spread.

Orion makes herbal tea. Zen and Callie cook pasta with pesto for dinner. The smells of good food and the pine tree fill the house. It all looks so normal, so cozy, as we gather around the fireplace. Tom and the boys play cribbage. The young women knit and watch me out of the corners of their eyes.

❊   ❊   ❊

The morning of Christmas Eve is the first time the house has been empty since I came home from the hospital. The sun sparkles on the lake between the bare trees. On the bird feeder, blue jays and cardinals, tufted titmice and mourning doves jockey for food.

With everyone out doing last-minute shopping, I wander into Tom's study and find a text on gyn oncology. When the phone rings, I'm thumbing through the index looking for the chapter on radiation for uterine cancer.

"They paged me," Tom says. "I'm at the mall. I've got the pathology report. Dr. Morgan rushed it, because he knew it was you."

I wait, expecting the worst. "So . . ."

"You're okay." Tom laughs. "Pats, you're going to be okay."

"What . . . what do you mean? There isn't any cancer?"

"No, there is. There *was,* but it was stage one, totally confined to the lining of the uterus, the endometrium. It was just a polyp. It didn't go through the organ at all, and the cytology washings were perfect. There were no cancer cells in your pelvis."

I lean back, staring at the oncology book in my lap. Brilliant sunlight floats into the white room.

"So what's up? You okay?" Tom asks.

I smile feebly. "Yeah, I'm fine. I'm great. It just feels weird after all the worry . . . I have cancer, now I don't. I was just sitting here reading about radiation therapy, and now I won't need it."

"I didn't think you would."

I'm standing up now at the window, looking down at the lakeshore, at the silver patterns shimmering in the ice.

I take a deep breath. This is too strange. I have to think about this. But I don't get to think about it. It's Christmas Eve, and the family comes home and acts as if we just won the lottery. Mica goes into the kitchen to break out a bottle of champagne. Even Orion's dog and our dog, Roscoe, get into the celebration, racing around the living room.

"What a great Christmas present!" everyone says. And it is. *It is.* The festivities swirl around me. It couldn't be better. I'm aware of the smile on my face, but it's only skin deep. I had cancer, now I don't . . . I fell through the roof of the world, now I'm dropping back in.

Outside the big windows, it's snowing again.

❈   ❈   ❈

Christmas is over. Then it's New Year's. Then the scurry of kids packing. There are hugs and kisses, wallets and keys to be found at the last minute. Tom loads the last of them into the Toyota and heads for the Pittsburgh airport. Orion, driving himself and Dozia home, will call to check on me tonight. Zen will call in a week. Mica will call in a month, but he'll feel guilty about it. That's how he is.

I gingerly walk around the house tidying up, putting cups and bowls in the dishwasher, wrapping paper in the trash, and dog toys in the basket, always with one hand on my incision. Tom will be gone for six hours.

When I can sit down without cringing at the mess, I make myself a cup of peppermint tea. Then, in the quiet, tidy house, I wait for the flood of feelings I've been too busy to feel. I stare out the window at the snow-covered branches, but nothing comes. No grief, no anger.

Since my emotions are apparently in hibernation and not available for reflection, I put in the Grateful Dead CD and start to dance, swaying to the rhythm, using my arms and hips more than my feet. *We will get by. We will survive.*

Then, since the cancer is apparently gone, I take my empty body to bed to see if it still works. I lie under the red and green quilt touching myself and am relieved to feel a faint motor purring. After another good long while, I'm able to climax. My female parts are gone, but I can still come! I'd feared the hysterectomy more for the loss of my sexuality than for potential complications. Tom had told me I would be okay, and he was right.

The sun shines down from the high window on my face. It lights the blue stained-glass mandala.

I sleep all afternoon, smiling.

CHAPTER 12

ARAN

On my first day back to work after the holidays and my two weeks of sick leave, I see Aran is an add-on at the end of the day, the reason for her visit listed only as *gyn problems*. I sit at my desk, checking my mail. Donna stops by. "How you doing?" she asks.

I shrug. "Fine. I guess everyone has heard the cancer is gone. They just scooped out my insides, washed up my pelvis, and *poof* —no cancer!" Donna squints, unsure what my sarcasm means, then leaves quickly.

I've thought about this appointment with Aran all day, wondering how it will go, wondering if I'll know what to say. Trish had called me at home three days ago to tell me Aran thinks she may have an STD. She also told me that Aran's not coming home at night. The girl leaves her baby, doesn't make any arrangements with Trish, and just disappears, doesn't say where she's going or when she'll be back. When she's not staying away from home she locks herself in her room. Trish is starting to wonder if her daughter is on drugs. I agree, this doesn't sound right.

When I enter the exam room at four, I find Aran sitting in her exam gown, her hands folded in her lap, looking as proper as a girl in a church choir, her short sandy hair shiny and clean, her face pale and without makeup. She wears nothing but thick green wool socks and the blue cotton gown, but she's thinner than I remember. Black combat boots are pushed under the guest chair. I decide to play innocent and see what she says.

"So how are *you*? I haven't seen you for a few months." I smile, staring into the girl's large blue eyes. It's hard to tell if the pupils are constricted.

"Not so good." The thin smile fades. "First of all, Jimmy and I broke up. I know we have before, but this is for real. I'm serious. For real. I took all my stuff and the baby's stuff too, and moved home. Now he has chlamydia, and I'm afraid I might too. I want to be checked for everything. He's such a dirtbag!" There are tears in her eyes, just floating on the edges, not flowing yet. She wipes them with a corner of the blue exam gown.

"So when did you last have sex with him?"

"Just a week ago. I thought we might get back together, but now it's *never* going to happen. I'll *never* forgive him! He's such a liar, and I stood up for him all this time, stayed with him at the hospital. I feel like a fool."

"You didn't use condoms, by any chance, did you?"

"No." Her eyes dart away.

After the exam, I have Aran sit up. "I've checked you for gonorrhea and chlamydia," I begin. "There's no discharge or redness. There are blood tests we need to get for HIV, syphilis, and hepatitis." Aran nods. "We'll have to wait for the results, but I want to say very seriously, *from now on you need to use condoms.* It doesn't matter how much you love a guy. It's *your* body. The birth control pills will only protect you from one thing—babies! And as you know, they're not even a hundred percent for that." I'm glad to see the corners of Aran's mouth turn up. The young woman got pregnant last time while taking the pill.

"I know," Aran says. "I really do know. And I *will*. I promise I'll use them. From now on, I will."

"There's something else," I continue. "Trish says you're staying out nights and not coming home. This concerns me, because I haven't seen a new mother act like this before. I know you love Melody, and I wonder if you think you could have postpartum depression or something." I'm winging it now.

"She *told* you?" Aran's steamed.

"Yeah."

"Well, I'm not using *drugs*. That's what they all think. My dad assumes I'm a crackhead." She laughs bitterly, the blue eyes blazing. "I'm practically the only one of my friends who isn't. If they only knew . . ."

"So how come you stay out all night? Don't you worry about the baby?"

"No, my mom will take care of her. She's real good."

I stop the questions for a minute, then go on. "So, do you think you could be *depressed*? You know, postpartum depression. Sometimes it starts months after the baby comes. Your life has changed dramatically, and there's been a lot for you to cope with. So many changes can wear a person out. Stress can make a person feel like running away."

Aran is staring at the posters on the bulletin board. "No, I'm okay. So long as I am with my friends, I'm fine." She's still turned away.

"What about when you're alone?"

Aran picks at her nails, which I notice are not as clean as they once were, and lets out some air. "I feel like crying. I just feel like crying all the time . . ." There's the *beep-beep* of the laser in the next room, but no other sound.

"So maybe it *is* some kind of postpartum depression."

Aran nods slowly, thoughtfully. "I've been thinking of getting out of here. Just loading up with the baby and going to my grandma's in Philly, but I don't have the money for gas, and my Escort's not in great shape."

I roll my exam stool closer. "I had postpartum depression once. At the time I didn't even know what it was, but I thought bad things. I even thought about *killing* myself. I don't know why. It wasn't like me. My life wasn't that awful really. Do you ever have thoughts like that?"

Aran sits up straight. "Killing myself? *No*, I could never do that. I think that this is the life God gave me and even if it hurts right now, everything happens for a purpose. I really believe that. I didn't want to have a baby. I never wanted to be a mom. I don't even like little kids very much. But I got one, for whatever reason. I would never kill myself. *I would never.*"

"That's good. I think everything has a purpose too, at least when you look at the *big picture*. Even if we can't see what the purpose is." We're both silent, staring at the cream linoleum tiles with specks of dark green.

I stand up and fill out a lab slip for the STD blood tests and write a script for antibiotics. "Do you think an antidepressant might help, Aran? I could give you some samples."

Aran shrugs. "I guess . . ." I can't tell if the girl thinks medication is a good idea or is just going with the path of least resistance, but she takes the two weeks of samples I give her and shoves them into her purse.

In a way I'm reassured. Aran's probably drinking more than she said and using *some* drugs, but maybe nothing heavier than grass. She may be depressed, but she's not suicidal.

"Will you come back to see me in two weeks?"

"Sure," Aran says, zipping up her pre-maternity size 3 jeans, "and thanks, Patsy." There's not a stretch mark on her beautiful body. "Thanks for seeing me. I was really upset."

I give her a little hug. Just a small one around her waist.

I'm surprised when Aran smiles widely, exposing straight white teeth, the kind that probably cost Trish a fortune at the orthodontist, and gives me a big hug back.

Loss of Faith

This is the last straw. I swear it is! Rebecca Gorham has finally replied to my e-mail and says that we have unfortunately underpaid our fall taxes by around fifteen thousand dollars. Okay, by $15,239. Now it's early January, for God's sake, and she's just figured that out! I've been sick to my stomach all day. Where are we going to get that kind of money again? She knows we don't have it. She should, anyway, she's the accountant.

Each quarter I've asked Gorham to get the IRS reports done on time so we don't end up short, and each time she has an excuse. Last spring she was dealing with her predecessor Robert Reed's screwed-up tax forms from two years before, a huge job and not her mess, so we didn't say anything when she was late. It's been less than a year since we dug ourselves out of the hole our pal Bob left us in. Then in late November, Rebecca went to Europe to visit her sick mother. How can you criticize that? And for Christmas, she traveled to Boston to be with her kids.

"Getting an extension is no big deal," she'd informed me back then. "Businesses do it all the time. I'll just fill out a form." Apparently the form never made it to the IRS office, and now there are additional penalties. This is not the most money we've owed, but the well's running dry.

I suck in a heavy breath. Tom finally agrees with me that we need to get rid of Rebecca, but when is the right time, and how shall we do it? The woman, though a disappointment, did work her butt off through the earlier crisis. Still, we have to get a new accountant, and soon. The trouble is, I no longer have confidence we'll make a good choice. We've been through this twice in the last three years.

It's three in the morning and I'm walking the floor again, carrying my jam jar of scotch. I wish we knew someone in business to guide us. When we'd finally gotten wise to Reed's shady deals, I received Gorham's name from a friend in my meditation group. Despite the glowing recommendation, Rebecca's been a bust; not as disastrous as Bob, but bad enough.

Tomorrow I'll ask the secretaries to call other physicians' groups in Torrington and find out who they use for accounting. If a name comes up twice, we'll interview him or her. We'll be expedient, but we won't rush into a decision this time.

I stand near the corner windows, staring into the night. The snow has drifted all day. Now the wind's picking up and it's coming down hard. And where will we get $15,239? There's just enough in the account to make payroll. Tom has already borrowed from his retirement fund to pay the boys' tuition.

Breathe in. Breathe out. Things will probably resolve happily. Tom says they will, anyway.

I lean back in the big white chair and curl my feet up. For a long time I rest there in front of the big corner window, watching the clusters of snowflakes shoot like sparks through the night.

KASMAR

As usual, I'm running behind in the clinic, but I stop short in the hall when a woman emerges from the restroom. She looks familiar, but for a minute I can't place her. Then it comes to me. It's Penny, the patient that picks.

The blonde's cheeks have a healthy pink glow. The pancake makeup is gone and the scars on her face have smoothed. "Hi, Penny," I say, studying the patient. She stands with her shoulders back, wearing a wine-colored sweater with slim black pants, but her blond hair is what strikes me. It's been cut short and curled, and the dark roots are gone. I hadn't seen her for months and I had truthfully forgotten about giving her the free microderm treatments. For a while we'd done them every two weeks. "You look good," I tell her.

Penny grins. "Thanks, I guess. I just saw the other nurse-practitioner for a yeast infection."

I want to ask more: *Have you stopped picking? Does your husband tell you how pretty you are? Who was the doctor that sexually molested you?* But the hallway isn't the right place. Nor the right time. "Well, I got to keep moving. You take care," I call out as I tap on the door of exam room 2.

"Hi, Kasmar." I plunk down on the stool. Running late again.

"You can call me Kaz." The patient's voice is lower now, and she has five-o'clock shadow on her square-jawed, freckled face.

"That's new," I say, meaning the name, not the beard.

"Yeah, like the sound of it? I introduce myself to colleagues and students now as Kaz Layton. Has a nice masculine ring." Kasmar's blue eyes twinkle and her voice goes up in a girlish way. I raise my eyebrows. She clears her throat and tries again. "Nice masculine ring," she repeats, an octave lower. We both laugh. When we first started treatments I was worried how the nurses and secretaries would react to the idea of our assisting a woman in becoming a man, but Kasmar's sense of humor has made her one of the staff's favorite patients.

"So, you feeling pretty good about everything, I take it."

"Yeah, I passed for the first time as a guy last weekend."

I glance at the dark gray Dockers-style pants, gray plaid shirt, and a red tie thrown casually over the back of the guest chair. On the floor are new men's hiking boots.

I push my stool back against the cool white wall and wait for the story. "Yeah?"

Kasmar turns sideways on the exam table and leans forward, her hands on her knees. Her brown hair is cut shorter each time I see her. This time it's shorter than Tom's. "So we were at that new seafood restaurant. You know the one by the mall? Jerry and I were having dinner." I nod. "And when the waitress took our order she called me *sir*. We almost lost it but I kept my voice low and ordered 'for the lady and I.' Seemed like a nice macho touch. 'Very good, sir,' the waitress said. That cracked us up.

"So dinner went fine. Their food's pretty good. But here's the great part. I had to go to the restroom, so I stood up and walked toward the back. As I got close, I was nervous. I hadn't given a thought to which john I would use.

"I just kept striding through the tables, wondering if anyone was watching me but trying to be cool. Finally, I saw the signs and almost turned back. There were two doors: one with a shark wearing a top hat and one with a dolphin wearing a dress." Kaz widens his blue eyes, clearly a guy now, telling this story. He wiggles his eyebrows.

"I look to see if anyone's watching." He swivels his head back and forth, acting it out. "Which one should I take? An elderly woman in a polka-dot dress comes out of the ladies' room and nods. I take a deep breath and go in with the sharks."

Kaz, the man, rubs the side of his face, feeling his two-day-old beard. "Yeah, it was a milestone." He grins.

I stand and give his arm an affectionate squeeze. "Hey, you're getting muscles! That's one of the side effects of the testosterone."

"Yeah, I'm taking some supplements and working out with weights too."

"That's great." I listen to his heart and lungs with my stethoscope. "The beard looks good. How 'bout everything else? You doing okay? Your labs are fine." I hand over the copy of the patient's results for cholesterol, testosterone, CBC, and liver enzymes.

Kaz grimaces. He stares at the sheet of paper without reading it, then hands it back. "I guess I'm okay, but not really. I've had some problems at home."

"You mean Jerry?"

"Yeah. She's having trouble adjusting to me being a guy. We were always a *lesbian couple*, see? We hung out with other gay women. Now what are we? A heterosexual couple? I don't think so. So who do we hang out with? Jerry misses her old *girlfriend*, Kasmar, but I want to be her *husband*, Kaz."

"Well, you're still with her, right? You're still working it out. You may have changed outside, but you are still *you* inside."

"Yes and no. I'm more confident now, more aggressive. I don't put up with bullshit as much, expect more respect from people I meet. And women are starting to come on to me." He grins suggestively. His straight teeth are even and white.

"Women? Really. Like what? When?"

"Oh, like at the agricultural conference I just went to in Syracuse. I had quite an entourage of female graduate students following me around." The smile fades. "But Jerry, she's still the love of my life. I don't know what I'd do if I lost her."

"Have you tried counseling? Maybe you're just in an adjustment phase. You have to admit, the situation is weird. I mean, to be in love with a woman who's turned into a guy."

Kaz snorts and rubs his beard again. "Yeah, we'll be okay. We have an appointment with our therapist next week. I'll tell you how it goes when I come back next time."

He stands up to leave. "We'll be okay," he says again, convincing himself.

I head for the lab. Did I do the right thing by helping Kasmar the woman become a man? I look back down the hall. As if sensing my thoughts, Kaz smiles and raises his hand in salute.

Mutiny

It's 4:35, the last patient's gone, and the staff is finishing up for the day. The receptionists file the labs, pushing the heavy sliding metal chart racks back and forth. I sit at my desk, staring bitterly at my last chart, running my fingers over its shiny yellow surface.

Our monthly meeting this noon had not gone well. The secretaries, nurses and practitioners, aware that we owe the Feds another fifteen thousand dollars, have voiced their concerns about the precarious future of the practice.

❀   ❀   ❀

"If you're going to have to close, you ought to tell us. Don't drag it out. We'll have to find new jobs. We have families," says Celeste. Her brown eyes single me out. I keep my face still but tighten my jaw. If I bite any harder I might crack a filling. Celeste doesn't look away. "You should have realized a long time ago that Gorham was worthless."

She's right, but Tom made decisions too, and yet somehow he's always *exempt* from such criticism. A few heads nod, agreeing with Celeste, all eyes on me. I study the women in their blue checkered uniforms, which we provide for them, a different color for every day of the week. We pay the best wages around. Granted, we are struggling, but where is the gratitude? Where's the support?

On the other hand, I reflect, they all have families. They depend on their incomes to make mortgage payments and keep food on the table. They have a lot at stake here too. They need these jobs. Celeste is just the only one with the guts to say it.

"If I were running this business, I'd hire an experienced office manager. Someone who knows what she's doing," Celeste goes on. I listen to her without expression, thinking that hiring an administrator would cost another forty-five thousand a year. Like we have that money!

❈   ❈   ❈

Though I resent being locked in the stocks before the whole village, I realize that there is frequently truth in hearing what you don't want to hear. I have my bachelor's degree in health-care administration, but I'm not an experienced CEO.

What hurts most is that while I was being publicly lashed, no one came to my defense. No one, not even Tom. What was he *thinking?* If my husband were the victim of this kind of flogging, I'd have backed him up. I was being blamed for all the practice's problems, while he sat picking his nails.

I should quit! What the hell . . . I brood for a moment then open the chart on the desk in front of me. When I think of the stories my patients tell me, my troubles always seem small. Like Rosa's story.

I push back my desk chair and stand, stretching my back. It's time to go home. Downstairs in the parking lot, most of the cars are gone, and the street lamps glow yellow. It gets dark so fast in the winter. I see Trish plowing steadily across the parking lot, her long blue coat blowing open, and I tap on the window, but it's four stories down. I know she won't hear me.

It's 5:15, and through my closed office door, I hear the staff joking as they clock out. Linda is clowning around. Apparently they have no idea how they hurt me. To hell with them all!

When their voices fade, I throw on my coat and scarf. Outside the wind has come up and it's raining hard. The roads will be icy, and the storm will be worse before I get home.

ROSA

Rosa's annual exam and wellness visit is going smoothly until, after reviewing her medications, I inquire, "You're taking both Xanax and Prozac? Is there a reason?"

"Is there a reason you need to know?" Rosa asks. Her dark brown eyes flash defensively. The fifty-year-old Hispanic woman I recognize as the secretary for the VP at the university hospital. Her smooth, unlined brown face belies her age.

"I guess, I just wondered because both medications will work for anxiety, but Xanax is quite addicting."

The woman takes a deep breath, looks down at her blue cotton gown, and then back up at me. "I might as well tell you. My son is in prison. He's in prison and every day when I think of him, I cry. He'll be there for ten years. No parole. I don't usually like to get into this."

"I'm sorry. It's okay if you don't want to talk about it."

"No, it's all right." The patient softens her low voice. "It's just that, how do I explain . . . He was an ordinary kid, a good kid. We're not this kind of family. Do you have children?" I nod. "Well, eight years ago, my husband had an affair with a woman in Delmont. To tell you the truth, it wasn't the first, just the most blatant. I got a divorce. I couldn't trust him again. I could never forgive him. I tried, but I couldn't. I just couldn't."

She clears her throat. "It was bad timing. Darren had just turned fifteen and began hanging out with the tough kids. He was living with me. One night he was beat up. I don't know who started it or what the fight was about. Some racial slur, maybe; he was sensitive like that. While he was in the ER they did a drug test. Turns out it was positive for marijuana and cocaine.

"They can't arrest you for testing positive. You know that. But it was a wake-up call. We tried counseling, and for a while Dee seemed to fly straight. We call him Dee, did I say that?" Rosa tells me all this as she stares at the wall directly behind me. I glance back, imagining a small TV screen with the marquee announcing the afternoon-movie feature: *A Mother's Nightmare.* "He was put on probation for the fight; they called it assault and battery, something like that, and he cleaned up his act. He had to be drug tested every week, but in less than a year he was picked up downtown, this time with marijuana *on* him. Somehow we got him out of that scrape. It was only a small amount of grass. They lengthened his probation, but gave him another chance.

"Then, a few years after he'd started college at State, it came out he was gay."

I swivel on my exam stool, close Rosa's chart, and lay it on the sink counter. I hadn't expected this turn in Rosa's story. "Gay?" I ask.

Rosa continues, "Yeah, but I was relieved about that. Everything made more sense. He's very good-looking, but his girls never lasted. Somehow, when he told us, I loved him more, but his father couldn't get over it." She takes a deep breath.

"And then Dee shot someone . . . He shot him, and the boy died. You probably read about that. Headline news in the *Torrington Tribune.* This was over a year ago now."

The story has twisted again in a direction I wasn't expecting. I rarely have time to read the *Tribune* and get most of my local news from Linda, who reads the paper each night.

"Dee was on cocaine," the patient tells me. "We know now that he'd been dealing drugs for some time. That's why he had so much money and so many new clothes. This other boy was in the process of breaking into his apartment to steal drugs when it happened. Darren was high and got scared. He pulled a pistol from under his pillow and shot the young man right in the chest. I don't think he'd ever fired a gun before, but what do we really know about our kids?"

I flash on the gun Tom found hidden in Orion's bedroom five years ago, a sawed-off shotgun. Tom was so pissed he ran down to the lake and threw it as far as he could. Orion denied it was his. Said he was just keeping it for a friend. What the hell were our boys doing with guns? We're pacifists, for God's sake! They'd been on peace marches before they could read! Rosa goes on with her story.

"At first Darren was freaked and hid out with friends, but in three days he turned himself in. We got a good criminal lawyer, Rock Durban. You know him?" I nod. I remember Mr. Durban. I know personally how good he is. He was our youngest son's lawyer when he was caught in the high school parking lot with ten little baggies of grass.

"Because of the break-in, the shooting was considered manslaughter and Dee was put on probation again. A lot of people in town were bitter about that, felt he should have been tried for murder."

"So if he got off, why is he in prison now? Did he violate his probation?"

"I guess you could say so. He got caught robbing a bank in Delmont with a rifle a month later." Rosa pauses. "He was high on meth this time. You see why I don't talk about this?" Our eyes finally meet. "It feels like someone else's life I'm describing. This can't be me. This can't be my boy. Anyway," she says, taking a deep breath, "there's no possibility of probation or parole. Armed robbery is a mandatory ten years in West Virginia."

For the first time there are tears in the woman's eyes. She wipes them at the corners with an actual hankie. "I'm sorry," she says.

"It's okay." I reach for her hand. It's cool and brown, white on the inside. "So, do you see him often?" I whisper.

"No. It makes me too sick. After I visit him in the prison I can't sleep; I cry all night. That's when I take the Xanax. I can't face him there, you know? I write him every week, but that's all I can do.

"He's just a beautiful kid . . . *man*, I should say. And so smart. He has his dad's height, but my coloring. He's clean now. No drugs in prison. But he's too beautiful. You know what I mean? He sold dope and had a gun, but I know him, he's not a tough guy. He'll be used. He'll be knifed or come out with HIV. If he learns to survive, he'll have to become member of a gang, a thug himself. Either way he's gone . . ."

We sit in silence. Rosa is thinking of her son. I think of my sons. Finally I stand and silently begin her examination. When I listen to her heart it is ticking away. *Lub-dub. Lub-dub.* I count the beats, eighty per minute. I would like to take her heart into my hands and hold it against my cheek. Not the real heart, you understand, the soul of the heart. The mother soul . . .

NILA

"Good, I *caught* you!" Abby whispers as she hurries down the hall toward me. "I've got to talk to you before you go in there." She indicates the exam room with a nod of her head and pulls me back into the lab. "Nila is back with irregular periods, and she's got a black eye, but don't say anything. You're not supposed to notice."

"What do you mean, *not notice the black eye?*" I counter. "Does Nila have makeup over it? How did she get it?"

"All she would say is, 'Just tell Patsy I don't want to talk about it.' That's all she said."

I close my eyes. I'm not good at ignoring something and keeping my mouth shut.

Nila was supposed to return in three months for a birth control check. It hasn't been that long. Hesitating for a moment, I knock my gentle greeting, tying to be casual. "Hi, Nila," I say as I enter.

The woman sits on the end of the exam table with her back to the door. "So, how are you doing?" I'm trying to be upbeat. "What brings you in today?" Nila's sandy brown hair, which she usually ties up in a ponytail, hangs down around her face. It's not just her eye. Her whole left cheek is mottled and purple. I make a quick assessment, then look away.

"The birth control patch wasn't working," the patient says flatly. "I spotted heavily for the first two weeks, so I took it off. Now I'm really messed up."

I glance again at the eye; messed up in more ways than one. "How much are you bleeding? Like a period?"

"No, I finally stopped, but it was real heavy for a while. I think I'm anemic."

"What makes you say that?"

Nila still hasn't made eye contact. "I'm just so tired. I can barely get out of bed. I figure I'm low blood, and the bleeding has caused it, first the miscarriage and then a period that lasted forever." She hunches at the end of the exam table, a deflated balloon.

I let out a breath. "Nila, I can't do this. Abby told me I'm not supposed to mention the black eye, but you think I'm blind? What's going on? The birth control problem is one thing, but you look like hell and you've lost weight. Is it Doug?"

"No, not Doug. It's Gibby."

"Did *he* hit you?" I'd forgotten about Gibby, the estranged husband.

"Not hit, really. He was trying to get in the house. While I was struggling to lock the door, he pushed it open and it bashed up my face. He's real sorry."

"Well, what was Gibby *there* for? What did he want?"

"Oh, he said he was there to talk, but I didn't want to. He's still sending flowers, trying to get back with me." I remember the small man, about five foot six, muscular, with a thick neck and blond hair that showed on his chest at the front of his open work shirt. He'd never come to prenatal visits but was at the births of their younger children.

"What does *Doug* say?"

"Oh, he was going to go after Gibby. He's a big man and could do some damage, but I said, Leave it be. Gibby didn't mean to hurt me. Now Doug's fed up. Says I shouldn't be talking to Gibby *at all,* that I'm leading him on. Says we should at least call the police again."

"Call the police *again?*"

"Yeah, we tried before but they didn't do anything. They said they couldn't make an arrest or set up a restraining order based on his making *threats.*"

"What do you mean, *threats?* Gibby has threatened you?"

"No, not *me.* It's Doug. He says he'll kill him."

I'm silent for a minute. This is out of my league. "So do you love Gibby? Do you want to be with him?"

"No, I love Doug, but he says Gibby's crazy, that he'll never leave us alone. He wants to go back to South Dakota, but I have the kids to think about. They just started school. Gibby will get over it once the divorce is final."

"You've filed for a divorce?"

"Yeah, I saw an attorney. I'm just hoping the black eye goes away by the next time I see him."

I shake my head. "Nila . . ."

"Gibby is not an evil guy, Patsy. He's just *upset.* I understand. We grew up together. You excuse a person you've known and loved for this long. You understand them. Doug is the one I'm worried about. He's not used to this."

We both study the floor.

"Well, let's get your periods straightened out. Maybe the patch isn't strong enough."

"No, I don't think birth control hormones agree with me. We'll just use condoms."

"But can you be real careful with condoms, Nila?"

The small woman crinkles her eye, her one good eye, then tilts her head. "I guess we'll *have* to."

I fill out a requisition for a CBC and thyroid labs to check the patient's blood count to see if she's anemic or has a thyroid disorder that would screw up her periods, then I reach into the cupboard over the sink and hand Nila a month's supply of multivitamins with iron. "Don't bother to cancel your other return appointment. I want to see how you're doing." Nila nods.

I don't just mean the woman's periods. I mean everything else.

CHAPTER 13

Money Changer

For once I've not relied on my husband or others to make a decision. I've found an accountant, Donald Collins, CPA, of Collins and Redman Financials. He's employed by five other medical groups in Torrington, and they all think he's great. Mr. Collins has already reviewed our quarterly tax statement and found three errors. The bill is now down to $11,341, which is still not small change, but better than fifteen thousand dollars.

It was hard firing Rebecca, but it's done. In cowardly fashion, we sent her an e-mail telling her that we needed an accountant who had more experience in health-care management. It was the chicken's way out. We never explained how disappointed we were with her. She shot a sharp e-mail back and warned that we'd be sorry for dropping her, but we held firm.

Donald has already met with us twice in the office. He understands our frustration at having no fiscal leadership and suggests that Tom take a temporary salary reduction until we catch up. I don't like it. My husband works hard, harder than many gynecologists who make far more money, but Tom agrees. He says he would rather earn less and have more peace of mind.

This evening after work, sitting near the corner window in the living room, staring at snow drifting sideways like feathers after a pillow fight, I wonder if we did the right thing when we gave up OB, but what choice did we have?

When the cost of medical-liability insurance almost doubled, we looked at what it would cost to continue obstetrics, and we couldn't break even. Bringing new life into the world in a gentle way was our calling, but a calling we could no longer afford.

JEANNIE

A quiet Saturday afternoon, with a cup of tea, watching the gray squirrels rob our birdfeeders. Seeing Jeannie Perry yesterday for her gyn annual reminded me of the *nonmonetary* rewards of delivering babies. The slender, dark-haired, thirty-six-year-old woman had been Tom's infertility patient. She'd been trying to get pregnant for five years and had been through all the tests, even surgery. She'd also tried artificial insemination with her husband's sperm three times, without success. Then the couple got pregnant on their own one warm spring night. Wouldn't you know it?

A year before we gave up our OB liability policy, we sent out letters to all our patients, telling them that as of January 1, we would no longer be doing deliveries. There were hundreds of women trying hard to get pregnant in the following months. Jeannie was one of them, and she just made our deadline. Her due date was January 3, three days *after* our insurance would be terminated, but we were counting on her going early.

As the holidays came and went, Tom and I waited for a phone call from Jeannie, but no call came. A few days before New Year's, I checked the young woman in the exam room and what I found wasn't good. The baby was head down, but Jeannie's cervix was closed. "Are you having *any* contractions, Jeannie?"

"Not many. I think something's wrong." Jeannie pulls her long straight dark hair back from her face.

"Yeah, can't you do something?" Nathan, her husband, mutters leaning forward in the guest chair. "It took so long to get this baby.

How many more days do we have wait for it to come out? What will we do if you can't deliver?"

I go over all the things I usually recommend to stimulate contractions—make love, take primrose oil, go on long walks—and then I sum up the situation. "If by December twenty-ninth nothing has happened, we'll admit you to the birthing center and give you a jump start. Sound like a plan? We won't let anything happen to your baby. Don't worry."

Saturday the twenty-eighth comes and goes. No phone call from Jeannie. Sunday morning. Coffee in front of the Christmas tree with Tom. (This was last year, before our IRS troubles, the gallbladder surgery, and cancer; before our little world blew apart.)

"So, Jeannie's coming into the hospital this afternoon," I remind Tom. "Today's the day . . . or tonight. One of us will have to go into town to admit her and get things going. I hate to tie up our weekend, but there are only a few more days left before January one."

He flips his warm palm over to hold my hand. "Let's both go. It's probably our last birth together. Call it a date. We'll get the induction started, then go to a movie. I've been nervous about this delivery all week." This catches my attention, and I wait for more. Tom's rarely anxious about obstetrics. "You heard what happened a few months ago to Dr. Gorday? Her last delivery before she retired? It was a disaster. The baby's head came out but the body was stuck, shoulder dystocia. She did a big episiotomy, cut almost down to the rectum, tried McRoberts' position with the woman's knees pulled back to her neck, tried the screw maneuver, even broke the baby's clavicle to get him out, but nothing worked. Gorday was shitting bullets. Finally had to do the Zavanelli procedure."

"The Zavanelli?" (All OB providers know about the Zavanelli. It's a last resort: you flex the fetal head, push it back in the mother's pelvis, and then do an emergency C-section.) "Did it work?" I ask.

Tom smiles. "Yeah, it worked. The baby was in intensive care for a few days, but he was all right. Now I understand Dr. Gorday's fear.

I was never scared before, but I just want to get this last one over. I have a weird feeling." The shadow of a hawk passes over the snow. I stand to look out the window but the raptor is gone.

By five on Sunday afternoon, Tom and I are sitting in an almost empty movie theater with a tub of popcorn and a Diet Pepsi. *Not much of a midwife,* I think, *watching a film instead of my patient,* but Jeannie was so totally comfortable after we'd placed the misoprostol in her vagina, I couldn't see the point of sticking around.

After dinner at our favorite Indian café and a short trip back to the birthing center, we go home to bed, fully expecting the nurse to call us in the middle of the night, but on Monday morning the sun rises and Jeannie's mild contractions have petered out.

It is high time to get serious, only two more days to go. I do an amniotomy early and start IV Pitocin, recognizing, with some discomfort, that I'm messing with nature, just so we can be the ones to deliver our patient's long-awaited baby. Then I settle down in the rocking chair to wait.

As the sun moves across the birthing room and shadows collect in the corners, Jeannie begins to moan. By six p.m., her uterine contractions are four minutes apart and moderate in strength, but her cervix is still only at three centimeters, *still* stiff and fibrous. Jeannie tries standing and swaying at the bedside, sits up in a chair, rocks on her hands and knees, but she's getting weary. "I don't care anymore about natural childbirth," she snaps at her husband when he tries to get her to do her breathing. "I want an epidural." No argument from Nathan. His wife's been a trouper.

At midnight, we switch. Tom settles down for the night in the doctors' call room, while I go home to our big king-size bed. Twice I wake and call the nurse for report, but at six in the morning I give up my effort to sleep and go back to the hospital.

When I walk into the pastel-wallpapered birthing room, Jeannie is snoring like an old man, poor thing; worn out. I nod to Tom, showered and dressed in clean blue scrubs, ready for the OR. "How dilated?" I whisper.

"Eight centimeters. I was up every few hours checking on her. The baby's fine. Should be out by noon." Always the optimist. I walk him to the doors of the surgical suite, where he's scheduled to perform a laparoscopy and two tubals.

At nine a.m., I help Jeannie wash up and braid her long hair. "Will we have the baby today?" she asks, her face pale with fatigue.

"Yep." (There are only fourteen hours until our OB privileges end. It *has* to be today.)

At eleven, Jeannie announces emphatically, "I need more pain medicine!" I glance at the monitor and pull on a sterile glove to check her cervix. "You don't need more medicine." I grin. "The baby's right here, ready to be born. It's time to push!"

So we push . . . And we push . . . For two hours, we push. It's a group effort.

We try every position the nurse and I can think of. "Can't we just do a C-section?" Nathan asks, eyeing the tracing as the fetal heart rate dips into the nineties, then bounces back to 150 again, a nice normal baseline. "Maybe he's *too big.*" That thought has crossed my mind too, but it's not time to give up yet.

"Come on, let's go back to work. We're missing some of these contractions. Here, Jeannie, pull on my hands. Pull!" An hour later, when Tom returns from the OR, he enters the birthing room as if he means business, and I'm glad to see him.

"How you doin'?" he asks Jeannie and shakes hands with Nathan. "Getting tired?" I catch his eye and glance toward the monitor. The decelerations are steeper now but always returning quickly to baseline.

Another big contraction and Jeannie grabs her butt then flops back in bed, trembling. "I don't think I can do this!" After two days of labor and three hours of pushing, the young woman is spent.

"Ready for some help?" Tom asks, slipping into a long green sterile gown. Terry, the RN, uncovers the delivery table and places a vacuum extractor, a modern alternative to forceps, near the corner. Clearly, *she* thinks it's time.

"You bet I'm ready!" says Jeannie. "Is this finally gonna happen?"

Though the extractor, which comes with a soft plastic suction cup, is less risky than metal forceps, it's not without danger. It can cause bruising, laceration, a hematoma, or worse, a shoulder dystocia, like Dr. Gorday ran into, in which the baby's head emerges but the rest of the baby gets stuck.

Dr. Harman parts the labia. "This may hurt a little," he warns as he applies the vacuum cup to the fetal head.

I center my attention. "Okay, Jeannie. Tom can't pull the baby out by himself. That would be too much strain on the little neck. You've got to push as hard as you can and soon you'll be holding your little one."

But I'm wrong. Each time Dr. Harman pulls, the head moves only a quarter inch. Once, the vacuum slips off. Then again it slips off. And again. The head is crowning now, and, by protocol, the provider gets only three tries with the extractor; any more may cause damage. Tom lays the mechanical device aside, then sits on the stool between Jeannie's legs, checking the vagina for stretch. Neither of us routinely does episiotomies—in fact, rarely, if ever— but I can tell he's thinking about it. Nathan stares numbly at the top of his baby's bruised head.

I reach over and pour a little oil, which the nurse has placed on the delivery table, over Tom's fingers as he massages the vaginal opening; our gloved hands touch and he smiles. Our last delivery together. Shoulder to shoulder.

When the monitor shows a good contraction, I lean over the bed and whisper to Jeannie, "This is it, babe! One more push. You're on your own now, no vacuum extractor. The head's almost out." With valor, the worn-out woman pulls back her legs once again. Nathan goes into position, holding her head, and I bend over, showing more optimism than I feel, to help Tom support the perineum.

Imperceptibly, there's a shift, and the fetal head dips below the public bone. There's no stopping Jeannie now. All at once, the baby rotates a quarter turn and hurtles into Tom's waiting hands. I place the wet squirming bundle in Jeannie's outstretched arms, cord still attached. "Thank you," she cries. "Thank you, everyone. My baby! My baby girl." Nathan is sobbing. There are tears in Tom's eyes. Our last delivery together.

I smile to myself now at the memory and take a sip of my peppermint tea, watching two scarlet cardinals, a male and a female, pecking around on the wooden bird feeder. Did we do the right thing by giving up OB? Are we better off now? A cloud crosses the sun, and Hope Lake turns gray. Then the clouds part again and the water is golden.

ARAN

Trish isn't at work when I call downstairs to family med to see if I can borrow some antibiotics for a patient that has no insurance and no money for medication. "Trish didn't come in," their nurse Cora tells me. "Give me a minute; I'll dig up samples and meet you on the back stairs." I trot down to the fourth-floor landing and greet Cora Jackson, a tall, lanky black woman wearing green scrubs.

"Trish sick?" I ask.

"Didn't you hear? Aran's in the hospital from a drug overdose. She was found behind Powell's Hardware, *clinically dead.*"

I go very quiet. "When did this happen? Yesterday?"

"No." She opens her eyes dramatically. "Sometime this morning, real early this morning, around four."

"Is Aran okay now?" I may look calm, but I'm sick with concern.

"She's lucky she didn't freeze to death. There was a heavy frost this morning. I had to scrape my windows. She was hypothermic, but she's stable. Some guy found her. He thought she was dead and called nine-one-one."

"But what was she *doing* behind Powell's?"

"Nobody knows. She probably won't know either. There are no bars around there, just some fast-food joints and a few little stores, but nothing open that time of night—well, morning. Maybe someone just dropped her off."

"Was it Jimmy? Could it be him?" I ask.

"Where you been, girl? Jimmy left the state. He got involved with some bad dudes and took off in a hurry. It was over drugs or something. I doubt he'll be back. Trish said he was going to clean his act up and join the army, but he'll be gone a long time."

"So, do you think some drinking buddies just dumped her?"

Cora shrugs.

I take the steps back upstairs slowly, thinking of Aran, thinking of Trish, my heart heavier than the forty-pound buckets of water I used to carry from the spring across the ridge to the cabin when we lived on the commune.

MARISSA

I glare at the last chart in the rack by the exam room door. I was hoping to get out early for a short bike ride, but it's not going to happen. Marissa Lewis, a new patient, is booked as a gyn exam but she's noted on the intake sheet that she has *many health concerns*. I take a deep breath, tap on the door, and reach out my hand. "I'm Patsy Harman, nurse-midwife and gyn practitioner."

The woman's cold fingers press mine. "I'm Marissa Lewis," she responds. Her dark-penciled brows give her a look of perpetual surprise and there's something fragile and strange about her. I'm thinking of white roses blown in the wind. Some of the petals are already gone. I go through my usual questions, asking about her reproductive health.

The patient is forty-four and menopausal, doing okay, she tells me, except for the night sweats and hot flashes. "They're horrible. I get wet all over. Sometimes I have to change my clothes twice before I leave home." She seems to accept the difficulty with good spirit, and laughs, but it soon becomes apparent that she's not well.

On the back of the patient-history form she's recorded her medical problems and surgeries. Five years ago, she had a total hysterectomy; afterward she experienced delayed healing and an infection. "It was awful. Now I have constant diarrhea. I go to a GI specialist at Torrington State University Medical Center. They say it may get better with time. And my pain is worse than it was before the operation." Marissa places her hand on her lower abdomen. "It's taken me a while to forgive the doctor. At first I thought of suing him, but what good would that do? I don't really know what he did wrong."

I squint at her medical history. Marissa has indicated that she sees an allergist, a cardiologist, a dermatologist, and an internist. She has joint pain and weakness. She's cold all the time and has allergies to eleven medications. She has skin sensitivity, rashes, and numbness of the tips of her fingers, not to mention the diarrhea and night sweats.

"Marissa, let's move on to the exam. Because you're attended to by so many other providers, I'm going to concentrate on your gyn health." I begin with the breasts and work toward her bottom. There isn't a lot to do. I assist the patient to rise. "Do you check your breasts monthly?"

"No, they hurt too much."

"Hurt all the time?"

"Just the skin. It hurts to touch my own skin, so I avoid it. Sometimes, even the air hurts my face." With the fingers of both hands, she circles her cheeks as if she's applying makeup. "Just the barest touch hurts."

The gesture's so eloquent. "Marissa, I know you're already seeing several specialists and I don't want to interfere, but you don't seem well. You have so many generalized problems. Have you been worked up for an autoimmune or a connective-tissue disorder?"

"Didn't I tell you? Didn't I write it down? I swear, I have brain fog. There's so much to remember." She rolls her light brown, almost golden, eyes to the ceiling. "It's one of my symptoms, forgetting things, like cotton was stuffed in my head. I've been to them all: Mount Sinai in New York, Johns Hopkins, and UCLA. That's where I finally got the diagnosis, at UCLA."

"The diagnosis?"

"Yes, fibromyalgia and—"

"Chronic fatigue," I finish. Now it made sense.

"Chronic fatigue *syndrome*," the patient corrects me. "It took years and a lot of tests and a lot of money, but we had to find out what was wrong. I was married then and had insurance. After the surgery, everything changed. I was a publicist in Pittsburgh and had lots of clients, writers mostly. I lost them all. I couldn't keep the pace. Then my husband left. He told me he hadn't signed up to marry an invalid. He thought I could snap out of it if I tried."

From my stool in the corner of the exam room, I listen as Marissa pours it all out, the pain, the worry, as she traveled from doctor to doctor. She stops her recitation. "I like your earrings."

I feel for my ears to see what I have on and touch my long woven silver links with blue beads. "Thanks. They're old. I stopped wearing such arty jewelry about ten years ago, but lately I've noticed it's back in style so I dug through my jewelry box and got them out."

"Oh, *very* in style." Marissa laughs.

Who is this woman? One moment she's talking about serious medical problems, the next moment earrings. "Are you married, Marissa?"

"I never know why doctors ask that. No. I'm single and happy with it." Her golden eyes sparkle and she raises those eyebrows. "Funny how sex helps with the pain."

"Really?" I ask. "It helps with the pain?"

"Yes, it does. I have much less muscle soreness after I make love. John, my lover, is very gentle. And here's something else. I tremble less after sex too. It seems to release something." She laughs. "I guess that's the idea, isn't it?"

I step out of the exam room to get a requisition for the patient's mammogram, and when I return, she's pulled on her sleek cream pants with an elegant wool stole draped over the sweater. "Nice outfit," I say. "You really do look radiant."

"Funny you should say that. You're not the first person. The more I let go of my anger about being sick, the better I feel. I've finally even forgiven myself for being weak, for being damaged."

I look at the petite, thin woman, in awe of her courage. Just thirty minutes before, I was in a hurry to get out of the exam room; now I'm reluctant to let her go. When she holds out her arms and hugs me, despite the difference in our sizes, I feel enfolded. She smiles and the room gets brighter.

"There really is something about you that shines, Marissa."

"It's the Lord," the patient replies. She picks up her engraved silver cane and steps out into the hall, then turns. "When all else fails, trust the Lord."

Weaver Dream

The full moon wakes me, shining through the high bedroom window right on my face. There was music, wind chimes, I think. There was a dream.

I sit straight up in bed, wondering what it could mean, and shake my head, struggling to understand. The red numerals on the alarm clock say 4:30 a.m. Through the window, I watch the clouds move fast across the sky. The full moon gives a false dawn. I remember then . . .

In a place of beauty, a forest carpeted with white trillium flowers, a woman sits at a loom. The wind flaps her skirt against her bare legs and she's weaving a tapestry of songs, fiber spun of scars, yarn dyed with tears.

This tapestry reflects faces I know: Trish and Aran, Holly and Heather, Kaz, Shiana, and Marissa. When the weaver is finished, she spreads the cloth on the earth and lies down. I see that my face is embroidered there too.

She closes her eyes and breathes deeply. The white bells of flowers sing her to sleep.

*

Spring Again

CHAPTER 14

KAZ

It's snowed all night, and patients are dropping out of the schedule like flies. As usual, the empty slots trouble me. Traditionally, this is a low month for billings, and we badly need money. I stand inspecting the list of appointments taped to my door. Three patients have already canceled. The next patient should be Kasmar Layton. He's never missed. Will he too call in? Outside my window, the thick wet flakes cover everything, a sloppy, wet spring snow, and the roads are too slick.

Kaz doesn't cancel. In fact, he comes early. I'm in the front office using the copier, and I watch though the glass over the receptionist's desk as he shakes the white off his hooded brown jacket and stomps his boots. His freckled face is red from the cold. If you didn't know different, he could be the FedEx guy delivering a package.

Later, in the exam room, after I've reviewed Kaz's labs, I sit on the stool and ask how things are. It's a slow day. I've got time to talk.

"Better," Kaz says. "Lots better. Things are settling down. Jerry and I have been getting counseling and feeling closer." He smiles. "Sex is the best it's ever been." Kaz goes on. "My only problem *now* is the faculty bathroom." Kaz's voice is low and doesn't have the adolescent breaks it did last time. His beard has thickened, and he's making an effort to dispose of the feminine gestures. I watch him, still amazed. Women can make their breasts large or small, slim down their thighs. We can alter our faces, smooth out wrinkles, lift drooping lids. We can even become men if we want to.

"So what's the deal with the bathroom? Last time I talked to you,

you'd used the guys' john in that restaurant and got a kick out of it. You told me you'd passed the test!"

"That was relatively simple, but last week I got a memo from the university that they don't want me to use the men's john in the agriculture building."

"Well, where are you going to go? The women's? I wouldn't think female students or faculty would be comfortable with that. I can imagine coming into the lavatory, seeing a guy like you at the sink, and walking right out again." We both chuckle.

"Exactly. That's what I told 'em." Kaz scratches his face.

"So, who's harassing you, the administration? The university lawyers?"

"Neither. Somehow the Department of Social Justice is involved. I think my chairman just didn't want to make a decision, so he handed it over to them. I never met more *unhelpful* people."

I frown. "So, what do *you* think the solution should be?"

"They should let me use the men's john and tell anyone who doesn't like it too bad!" Kaz grins. "Or build me my own bathroom. The chairman has one."

"Is there anything *I* can do? You know, write a letter saying that it's medically necessary for you to urinate on a regular basis or you'll have bodily harm?" I think this is funny, but Kaz doesn't smile. There's a pause. "Everything else okay?"

Kaz shrugs. "No big deal. Enrollment for my classes is stable. I mostly work with grad students anyway, but I'm not getting fan mail. Actually, I've been getting hate mail every day, e-mails and snail mail, obscene. I don't even want to tell you what the letters say. I'm sure the persecution is coming from only a few people, but my skin isn't as thick as I thought it would be. I keep looking around at faculty and students, wondering who it could be."

I watch Kaz, watch the tears hang on the edge, and I wonder what kind of courage it takes to go from a woman to a man in front of your colleagues. He wipes the tears away with the back of his hand, which has hair on it now. Moving out of state, starting fresh in a new community where the professor could pass for a male from the start, would be so much easier. "I'm sorry; I guess I never thought how that could hurt. How can you help being bitter? You never did anything to them. Do you have people to talk to who've been through this?"

"I'll be okay. It doesn't help to be angry. I just let it go. Anyway, I have the support group at the Persad Center. I'll probably start going to meetings again. I'll be okay."

"There aren't any *threats,* are there?" I'm worried for my patient's safety. This could get ugly. What if something happened to Kaz, like those incidents of gay-bashing you read about? I could never forgive myself.

Kaz smiles. He sees where this is going. "No threats. Just harassment. Don't feel responsible. I knew it wouldn't be easy. I could report the letters to the Department of Social Justice, but they wouldn't be sympathetic. You see how they are about the bathroom. I've made the *choice* to become a man. This kind of discrimination isn't like skin color or a disability. Anyway don't worry . . . I'm making muscles." He squeezes his biceps and hits his chest a few times like Tarzan. "I'll fight them all off!"

This time I *do* hug Kaz. I feel his back under my hands, harder, heavier, and probably hairier.

LEVY

At four, Noelle, our quiet billing specialist, comes into my office looking sober and closes the door behind her. "Do you know anything about an IRS levy on our Accordia reimbursements?" Her normally pale face is whiter than usual and tight around the mouth. "I just discovered, while finishing the monthly report, that we haven't been getting our West Virginia Medicaid payments. When I called the regional office in Charleston, they told me they've been withholding our money for months at the Internal Revenue Service's request. They're always so slow in paying . . . I didn't realize. Apparently, that's why our cash balance is so low. They're holding over twenty thousand dollars." She gives me a faxed correspondence with a shaking hand.

I'd seen something about this before Christmas, a warning letter that we were behind in our taxes and that our account could be attached, but I thought they meant the business bank account. I'd never dreamed they could take away our insurance reimbursements! Rebecca Gorham had said it was an error and that she would take care of it.

"This is a mistake," I reassure Noelle. "We don't owe them twenty thousand!" I toss the fax from Medicaid into my in-box. "We do owe eleven thousand for last fall's quarterly taxes, but we still have two weeks to pay. I'll have Don Collins straighten this out tomorrow," I say calmly. "Don't worry about it." Noelle looks doubtful but turns to go back to her desk. As soon as she leaves, I frantically shoot off an e-mail to our new accountant.

Don: We just heard from West Virginia Medicaid today that they've withheld $20,000 of our reimbursements because of some IRS levy. A letter came through from the Internal Revenue Service a few weeks before we hired you, referring to this, but Rebecca said it was a mistake and she'd take care of it. How can they take our money? We only owe the Feds $11,000 for the late fall taxes, and we're not even to the deadline. I'm freaking out: $20,000! Please call me. P. Harman.

I'm drowning in a net of levies, attachments, extensions, low bank accounts, and loans. I'm a good swimmer, but I'm going down! With all my concerns about the IRS, I realize I've neglected to call Trish. Her daughter almost died, and all I'm thinking about is money.

SHIANA

"You've got to come right now," says Donna, standing at my office door. "There's a girl out here that's having a fit." I have no idea what I may find, a belligerent or mentally ill patient or a young woman having a seizure. The receptionist pulls me by the sleeve around the corner, but there's no patient. "They must have taken her into an exam room," says Donna.

Running down the back hall, we find a small woman lying on her side on the floor of room 1. Celeste is trying to rouse her. The patient moans. Thank God, she's still breathing. No need for CPR. Though we're all trained, we've never had to resuscitate anyone. "Let's turn her over. Can you get her blood pressure?" I reach for the pillow. When I turn back, I'm shocked to see a pink baseball cap on the cream tile floor. It's my young patient Shiana. The girl with the blue condom.

"I'm so hot," the patient moans.

"Shiana, honey. It's me, Mrs. Harman. Are you okay?" Her light brown skin is clammy. A tall blonde with an overbite stands in the corner, clutching a cell phone. She wears tight black leggings and a gray sweatshirt with the same Greek letters as the pink cap. "Are you her friend?" I ask.

"I'm her sorority sister, but I *am* her friend, her *good* friend," she says, as if fearing I'll ask her to leave.

"Can you tell me why she's here today?"

"She's been real sick. She was in the emergency room last night with an ovarian cyst. Dr. Harman was going to do surgery tomorrow. We were about to go to the hospital to get pre-admission testing when she said she had to lie down. I thought she was going to collapse right at your checkout desk, but the nurse and I dragged her in here. We were trying to get her on the exam table and she slid to the floor."

The patient is mumbling.

"Sweetie, can you sit up?" I ask. "Shiana, honey . . ."

The girl shakes her head no.

Celeste returns with a cool cloth and the blood pressure cuff. "Dr. Harman is already at the hospital," our LPN tells me. "I hate to see her lying on the floor. Can we move her? Is she in pain? Maybe the cyst burst."

"Floor feels good," the patient says. "It just feels good. Cool." Her blood pressure is 80/40, too low, and her pulse is tachycardic, way too high, 120.

I turn to the friend, who still stands flipping her cell phone open and closed, ready to call someone but not sure who. "Do you think she hit her head when she fell? Do you know if she has any history of seizures?" The girl shakes her head no to both questions.

A voice comes from the floor. "I'm just so weak. I can't sit up."

"We'll let you rest then. If you feel better in about ten minutes we'll take you in a wheelchair across the street to the hospital. If you don't, we can call nine-one-one. You stay with her, Celeste. I'll tell the other nurses you're in here." When I come back ten minutes later, they're gone. Celeste has taken her to the emergency room. Celeste doesn't need much instruction.

That night, I hear more about Shiana, but the news isn't good. Before dinner, I page Tom to ask his estimated time of arrival. A circulating nurse tells me Dr. Harman's still in the OR. It's been over two hours.

Shiana had been added to the schedule as an emergency case, but Tom should have been home by now. If she'd just had a simple cyst on her ovary, why would the surgery be taking so long? Ever since Dottie Teresi's prolonged hospitalization, I worry about the slightest surgical problem.

I take my cup of chamomile tea out on the porch and rest my head on the railing. There's the scent of dirt and new things growing. The ice on Lake Hope creaks, shifting in the thaw. Then a crack like a gunshot cuts through the night as a chunk breaks away out on the cove. A few minutes later Tom walks through the door, whistling. It's eleven at night, and he's been on his feet since six a.m.

"What happened?" I ask anxiously. We both know what I mean, but he's looking like a cat that's enjoyed a bowl full of cream. He holds out a digital photograph taken through the laparoscope.

"It was really something. There wasn't just a large ovarian cyst. When I got in there, her ovaries and fallopian tubes were inflamed and swollen. Her uterus was enlarged too. At first, it looked like cancer, but when I saw all the pus . . ." He stares down proudly at the photo of his handiwork. I can't figure out why he's so pleased.

"PID?" I ask. "Pelvic inflammatory disease?"

"Yeah, infection all through her pelvis. There was nothing else I could do, I had to take a seven-centimeter cyst off, take down the adhesions, and irrigate the whole pelvis. She'll be in the hospital for a few days with triple IV antibiotics but she'll be okay."

I remember Shiana lying on the floor of the exam room. She must have been close to septic shock, bacteria already coursing through her bloodstream, shutting her organs down. "I guess we'll have to notify her parents in Erie," I worry aloud. "Remember, she's the girl I told you about, the college student who came in with the condom left in her vagina. Since then, she's had herpes, chlamydia, a yeast infection, and now PID. Her parents don't even know she's sexually active, and all this came about from that one condom accident."

"Oh, they're already at the hospital. Her friend must have called. I stopped by the waiting room and talked to them after surgery."

"What did you tell them? What did you say? You didn't tell them about the STDs, did you?"

"They're fine. They think the infection came from the cyst, and I didn't elaborate. Her folks are just glad she's alive."

Tom is exhausted and falls right to sleep. For a while I lie in the dark thinking about Shiana. Then my mind shifts to Medicaid withholding our payments. With the worry about Shiana's collapse, I hadn't told Tom that the Feds have twenty thousand dollars of our money. Maybe I should have called the IRS myself, months ago, when we got the letter warning us that our bank account could be levied for late tax payments, but I was facing cancer then and Rebecca had assured me she would take care of it.

Tom rolls on his back and starts snoring. I poke him. "Tom." I poke him again. "Tom . . . you're snoring."

"Okay," he mumbles and turns back on his side. In a few hours he will start snoring again. He does this when he's exhausted.

Outside the high window, the silver moon slips through the feathered clouds. I pray that the pelvic inflammatory disease won't make Shiana sterile. I pray that she won't get an abscess, like Mrs. Teresi, or chronic pelvic pain syndrome, like so many of our patients. For now she's okay. She survived being septic and lived through a complicated surgery. I just hope she will survive the emotional trauma.

In the dim hospital room, her parents keep watch at her bedside. I picture a vase of pink roses on the windowsill. The father, a big man, sleeps soundly with his bare brown arms hanging over the edge of a narrow fold-up cot. The mom, wearing the pink baseball cap over her dark curls, is still awake, sitting in the beige guest chair. She reaches over and tenderly places the back of her hand on Shiana's brow, checking for fever, as mothers do, as Trish has done for Aran, and Holly's done for her daughter, as I have done for my boys.

My husband starts to snore again. This time I let the poor guy be. I remember what Tom said one time: "I like being a surgeon. I like fixing people. It makes me happy."

Blame

Tonight Tom and I had a royal fight, and we've gone to bed mad. It's too bad. We'd had a great bike ride, our first one this spring.

Bluebonnets bloomed at the side of the path. The green river moved along on the right, and the sky rippled with clouds like the scales of a fish.

Later at home, sitting on the porch in the dark with our peppermint tea, I cautiously bring up the office finances. For weeks, Tom's been too tired or preoccupied to talk about our situation. He's off to the hospital at six in the morning and not home until nine at night. His face is blotchy, with scaly patches of eczema. He's literally working himself sick to make money. He says I dwell on the problems, but someone has to.

For the first time in months, I sleep alone in my study. Not that I'm sleeping. Don Collins called this morning to confirm that Noelle's information is correct. The IRS has, in fact, been withholding our money. All payments from West Virginia Medicaid and PEIA state employees' insurance have been withheld and will continue to be withheld until the agency receives verification that we've paid our taxes. Meanwhile, even though we owe only eleven thousand dollars, they continue to withhold more of our money. And it's worse than Noelle thought, not just twenty thousand but *thirty-three thousand dollars!* Don has filed an appeal with the IRS but says in his experience it will take months, possibly years, to get it all back. The Feds have no record of Rebecca ever requesting an extension for the fall quarterly taxes.

Our financial problems are not really Tom's fault, and I know that, but I don't understand how this happened. He has the office accounts on his computer. Couldn't he see that our balance was crashing? Tom thinks I'm responsible. As the practice administrator, I should have followed our insurance payments more closely. Really, we're both just scared.

There's four hundred dollars left in the checking account, and staff salaries yet to pay. The eleven thousand is due in a week, and we're still not clear where we'll get it. Don has suggested we go back to the bank, but we owe so much money already. The practice debts are guaranteed by a mortgage on our home on Hope Lake. If the business goes down, Tom and I will lose everything. Maybe it would be for the best. We could start over, go back to being hippies. I smile wryly and let out a long sigh, picturing us out on a farm in the hills, chopping wood, carrying water, canning and drying our homegrown crops. Outside my study window, there's nothing but blackness and the shadow of the red-leafed ornamental plum just budding out. No moon, no stars.

All day, Noelle has been on the phone trying to collect patients' past-due accounts, her black hair knotted at the back of her neck with a rubber band and a pen stuck into the knot. The staff knows what a mess we are in. Donna at checkout is insisting on payment at the time of service. Linda is calling patients with outstanding bills; some still owe us thousands of dollars. Everyone is doing what she can, but I'm afraid the bank will deny us more credit and I feel like a fool even asking them. If we can't manage our finances better than this, why would they trust us to pay the loan back?

I think of crying, but what good will that do? I turn the light out and reach for the jam jar of scotch, imagining Tom sleeping soundly in our spacious bedroom in our big, soft king-size bed while I toss and turn on this narrow cot. He's in the OR again in the morning and on call at Torrington State University Medical Center tomorrow night.

There's no getting around it, and there's no other choice. I can't wait for my husband, and I can't put it off any longer. I'll call the bank in the morning.

❊   ❊   ❊

The forecast for today is for partial sun, but there's no sign of it yet. For six days it's rained, and the lake as I cross the bridge is shit brown. Gray skies, brown lake, that's my life. All night I've been worried about the staff meeting. Tom, as usual, has slept like a log.

Though getting the loan wasn't as hard as I thought, it's only a stopgap to pay off the quarterly taxes and get us through another pay period. Don has told us straight out that we're spending more on overhead each month than we earn. He suggests that Tom and I cut employee benefits to save money, but it's hard. Both our fathers were union men, and we feel a sympathy for the workers. These benefits are part of the package they signed on for.

We've finally agreed, as a compromise, to cut back our contribution to their 401(k). As Mr. Collins points out, no other doctor's office contributes nearly as much as we do. If the business goes under, the staff will be out of their jobs. A cushy retirement fund won't mean much then. Don has promised to come to the meeting for support. I'll need it. I still burn from the harsh words directed at me at the meeting a few months ago.

At four, we close early and gather in the waiting room, where there are enough chairs for everyone. The atmosphere is as cloudy inside as out. Nobody says anything. Abby stares at the large framed photographs of pink magnolias. She has to go to her mother's farm outside Helvetia this weekend. Her mom's slowly losing her mind, and Abby desperately needs to hire someone to stay with her, even if she has to pay for it out of her own pocket. Usually bouncy Linda gazes out the long windows at the dark clouds. Her husband is still out of work at the mines. Now her paycheck is all that they live on. The rest of the secretaries and nurses sit waiting, no joking, no gossiping. Then everyone turns toward the door.

When Donald walks in with his briefcase in hand, I'm sure they're expecting the worst. I, as usual, play master of ceremonies when everyone gets settled, too anxious to keep quiet and give my husband an opportunity for leadership. "We've asked Donald Collins, our new accountant, to join us today to give everyone an overview of the practice's financial picture." Tom slumps in his chair, staring down at his shoes, while I babble nervously on. He's still wearing his scrubs from the OR.

"I know some of you have been concerned about the money picture for the practice, and this meeting will give everyone an opportunity to ask questions."

Donald pulls a ream of paper out of his briefcase. "How's everyone doing this afternoon?" he asks cheerfully, a ray of sunshine in the gloom.

He summarizes our situation: "The practice is spending more than it makes and is gradually going deeper and deeper in debt. In addition, the IRS has instructed several government insurance plans to withhold your payables, and that has hurt your bank account significantly. I've come up with some recommendations." All eyes are pinned on his face. "I've told Patsy and Dr. Harman that, while I respect their generosity to their employees"—he looks around the group to be sure everyone is listening—"it's part of the practice's financial problems.

"Since Dr. Burrows resigned and you dropped obstetrics, what you collect isn't equal to what it costs to do business. Now, there isn't any way to cut most of that expense. The rent for the office, supplies and so forth, are fixed. To make up the deficit, we could cut staff or health insurance benefits." People shift in their seats uncomfortably. "Or we could cut salaries." A telephone rings, but no one gets up to answer it.

"The Harmans have insisted that they are unwilling to do this." If there was a bomb in the room, we'd hear it ticking. "What we've decided to do instead is to drop the employer's part of the retirement contribution from the ten percent they've contributed in the past to the three percent that's required by law." He pauses to let that sink in. Collectively, the group lets out a long breath.

"Originally, Dr. Harman explained to me, the ten percent was a way to share profits with employees, but for the last few years there haven't been any profits. Dr. Harman has, in fact, taken a considerable salary reduction this year to keep the business afloat." I hold my breath, waiting for the staff's reaction. It feels like the moment in a dive before you hit the water. You know it will be cold, but you don't know how cold.

Celeste speaks up. "Well, I think this is sensible! It's not what we want, of course, but if it keeps the practice going, I'm all for it."

The women murmur agreement. "I'm sorry about Dr. Harman's salary though." Everyone turns to Tom, who stares at the hunter green carpet. I know he feels bad about the 401(k) cuts. I feel the same way.

"Hopefully, next year will be better," Donald continues. "Once we get the taxes caught up and the practice stable, we can consider contributing more to your retirement fund." I find it comforting, the way he says *we*.

My husband clears his throat. "I just want to say that it's okay about my salary. I don't want anyone to feel bad about it. Patsy and I could always use more money, with the boys in college, but I can use the peace of mind more. Knowing we can pay the bills here without difficulty will take a lot of weight off me." He doesn't say anything about the second mortgage on the house we've just had to take out in order to make the looming IRS payment.

"Any questions?" Don asks. No one speaks, so, with a rustle of papers, Don stands and begins to pack up his briefcase.

Tom hurries out to make rounds in the hospital, and the nurses and secretaries disperse cheerfully, happy that no one will be let go, they'll each continue to get a paycheck, and they'll still have their health insurance.

"Thanks, Don," I say, leaning over to touch his veined hand as he puts on his raincoat. "You made that much easier."

As Donald Collins goes out the door, he salutes me with a twinkle in his blue eyes, my smooth, mild-mannered accountant, man of steel, our hero.

TARA-SUE

I nudge Tom's arm and point down to the lake. "Did you hear that?" He cocks his head. "Peepers. I think it's the peepers." We sit silently in the dusk on the side porch, sipping mint tea, but the high ringing sound doesn't come again. There's no sound but the trucks on the distant freeway.

"Early yet," Tom says. "Too cold."

I don't think so. I'm sure that I heard them. It's Friday evening and the air smells like wet dirt. He's been in the OR since early this morning.

"Can I tell you a funny story? I've wanted to tell this to someone all day." Lately my husband's been so tired and moody I've been overly polite. I never know what to expect from him, and we still haven't gotten over the fight about the IRS levy, never apologized even, just went on as if nothing had happened. When I hold hands with him there's no song in our touching. I'm getting so I hardly care.

"Sure." Tom puts his feet up on the porch rail. Beyond us there's nothing but green. The green locust that grows close to the front porch hangs with white grape-like blossoms, the green lawn on the side, the green peach trees and tall ash and pines. West Virginia in spring is the green of Ireland. The sky in spring, however, is gray. The gray of sidewalks and ashes and shadows, a dripping-wet gray.

"Well, this morning," I begin, "as I passed through the waiting room I see this slim middle-aged redhead, you know the type, classy, with nice legs and sling-back sandals. She had on a flashy lime twin-set sweater with a low-cut V-neck. I couldn't help noticing. Push-up bra and everything. Ten minutes later she's in my exam room, wearing nothing but the blue exam gown and these huge silver hoop earrings. I mean *huge,* you could have worn them for bracelets.

"So I ask her the usual questions and proceed with the exam . . . You still listening?"

"I'm here."

For a second I think I hear peepers again, but then they're gone, so I continue.

"Well, get this. I'm just starting the pelvic when her cell phone rings, some catchy salsa tune. She flings herself off the table. I'm not kidding. She grabs the phone out of her huge handbag and says, 'What do you want? I'm kind of busy right now.' I stand waiting with my exam gloves on.

"'Well, for God's sake! Do you know where I am? At the *gynie office.*' She has a kind of nasal twang, Dolly Parton with a stuffed-up nose, a breezy good-humored way of talking. 'Well, tell him I'll call as soon as I'm done.' She slaps the phone shut, rolls her eyes, and hops back on the table.

"I'm adjusting the exam light, getting ready to start again. 'Sorry,' she says, 'that was work. If I'm out of contact for a minute they have a crisis. It's a bunch of men. None of them cute!' She lies back, putting her feet in the footrests, and spreads her legs as if she does this every week. Then the salsa music on the cell goes off again. She jumps up like before, grabs the cell phone, and gets back on the exam table and lies down again. She looks at me and waves me on, like I'm supposed to continue the exam while she talks. I hesitate for a minute, thinking, *This is bizarre,* and then do what she says. I can't wait all day."

"You examined her while she talked on the cell phone?" Tom chuckles.

"Yeah, this is a first, and you should have heard the conversation. Apparently it was the guys at work again, International Fish or something. 'What now?' she snaps. 'What's the big hurry? More lobster? Didn't they get the first shipment I had flown in? Okay, put him on.'

"Now she tries to move the phone to the other ear and it gets stuck in her big hoop earring. I'm not kidding. She's fooling around with her cell phone while I'm doing her Pap test.

"'You *know* where I am,' she goes on. 'My *gynecologist.* I'm on the exam table . . . For real . . . Yeah, right now.' She tells some customer this, winking at me. I think she enjoyed shocking him. 'Well, just remember the next time you see my district manager. Tell him I'm such a good rep I even take client calls during my gynie exam!'

"By this time I'd finished and was taking my gloves off. She bounces off the table and starts to get dressed. I'm just standing there with my mouth open.

"'I take it that was an emergency?' I say finally.

"'Yeah, a lobster emergency. This resort in Laurel Springs has a big party coming in and needs thirty lobsters tonight.' Then she steps into her high-heeled sandals, gives me a wave, and is gone."

"A lobster emergency," Tom repeats. "That's a good one."

I watch him out of the corner of my eye, wondering if he thought it was as funny as I did. He's in a good mood tonight, tired, but relaxed. It helps that we got the loan and paid off the Feds. Don's leadership with our finances has relieved another burden. Now if we can just get back what the IRS stole from us, if we can just catch up . . .

Our eyes meet. I know what he's thinking.

"Want a glass of wine?" he asks.

Why not?

CHAPTER 15

ARAN

At seven on Monday evening, as I'm getting ready to take the dog for a walk, the phone rings. I tuck the receiver under my ear and try to continue tying my running shoe. "Hey," I say, expecting it to be Tom. It isn't.

Trish is sobbing into the receiver. "Aran, she's . . . she's gone. Oh, God! Aran! Aran . . ." The rest of the sentence is garbled.

"Aran's gone? Trish, slow down! I can't hear you. She's *gone?*" I can't understand her. "Did you say she took the baby? She took Melody?" Adrenaline is shooting through my body, and I feel like someone has punched me in the gut. "What's happening?" Trish takes a deep breath, trying to get it together. "I'm sorry. Aran's gone. I mean, she's *dead.*"

The colors all change in the room and I sink down on a dining room chair, almost knocking it over. "She's dead. No, she can't be!"

"I know. She can't be, but she is." Trish sobs

I feel faint and put my head down. I'd just seen Trish in the parking lot a few days ago and everything was fine. Well, sort of fine. There must be some mistake.

"What happened? You have to tell me. Breathe."

There's the muffled sound of a nose being blown. "On the way home from work tonight I called Dan on the cell to say I was going to pick up some groceries, to tell him I'd be a little late. He told me, 'Forget it. Just come now.' So I did. The sheriff's car was in front of our house.

"As I pull into the drive I'm wondering, *What's Aran done now?* But when I walk through the door, I see Dan crying, sitting on the sofa holding Melody. He tells me to sit down, and it just feels all wrong." Trish is almost whispering. "But I never expected this . . ." She trails off, then starts up again. "Oh, Patsy, I know I said it the other day, that she'd end up dead or in prison, but I didn't mean it . . .

"And the sheriff says, 'I'm sorry to tell you, ma'am, that your daughter was found dead this afternoon in her trailer.' Just like that. *'Your daughter was found dead.'* Her girlfriend Leslie discovered her and tried to wake her up but couldn't. 'I'm sorry to tell you, ma'am,' that's what he said."

I picture a pretty girl shaking Aran on a bed in a run-down trailer. *Wake up, silly! It's two in the afternoon. Let's go get some burgers. Let's party.* Leslie shakes the limp body harder. *Come on, Aran . . . rise and shine . . . Baby? . . . Honey? . . . Come on!* She's getting scared.

"So Leslie ran to the neighbors'," Trish says, clearing her throat, "and called nine-one-one, but it was too late." It's quiet for a few seconds, then our voices begin to run over each other's, both saying the same thing in different words. "Oh God, our kids are supposed to grow up and grow out of it."

"It can't be true."

"Oh, Aran!"

"Oh, Trish!"

Then finally, "I'm sorry. I'm just a mess. I just wanted you to know."

I'm still sitting at the dining room table, holding on to one shoe and clutching the phone like it's Trish's hand.

"It's okay," I say. "You can't help it. This isn't supposed to happen. You did everything you could."

"I want to turn back the clock. I want this to be yesterday and she's still alive," Trish says.

"What can I do?" I'm standing now, ready to bolt out the door.

"Nothing, I'll be okay. I just wanted to tell you . . . They've already taken her to the morgue in Charleston for an autopsy. The cop wouldn't say what happened, but it was a drug overdose. I know it. He said they'd confiscated some pills, but there was no evidence of violence or foul play." Trish begins to cry again. "I didn't even get to say good-bye. I didn't get to say good-bye or even see her before they took her away."

"Oh, Trish. You want me to come over and take care of Melody? What can I do?" I ask it again.

Trish blows her nose. "Nothing. We're going now to get Aran's stuff. Our neighbor is taking Mellie and the kids."

"Where did she live? Where are you going?"

"Glen Terrace. It's that trailer park by the old power plant, out Hadley Road. She'd just moved back there with Leslie a few weeks before she was found in the alley."

"You want me to come? I'll come too . . . You sure you want to do this now?"

"Yeah, I have to. I have to see. I'll be okay."

"Let me know if I can do anything, Trish . . . I love you." I'm startled. I've never said this to Trish before. I'm still holding my shoe, and Roscoe is sitting there looking at me, with her leash dangling from her collar.

"I love you too," Trish says.

※　　※　　※

Hadley Road runs for only two miles between the airport and Crocker Creek Bridge, but I can't find Glen Terrace anywhere. Though Trish told me not to come, I have to be with my friend.

A thick fog is pouring into the hollows, and I take a road down behind the adult video store when I see a few trailers, but there's no trailer park. I almost run the Civic into a ditch. *Slow down,* I tell myself. *Keep it together.* I'm gripping the steering wheel so hard my hands tremble. I want to find Trish, want to hold her, want to smother her pain with my body.

I head back up Hadley going the other way, and cut behind the Methodist church. In the parking lot, I call Tom on my cell phone. "Hey. Where are you?"

"Just leaving the hospital. Where are *you?*"

"I'm near the Glen Terrace Methodist Church. I've got some terrible news." I don't know how to say it nice, so I just say it. "Aran was found dead this afternoon. They think she died of an overdose. Trish just called me. She and Dan are going to her trailer to pick up Aran's things. I don't know why they have to go now, but the cops have already taken Aran to Charleston for an autopsy, so I guess Trish just needs to see where she died. I was trying to meet them but I can't find it."

Tom stops me. "Aran's dead?"

"That's what I've been saying." I take a shaky breath. "I've been up and down Hadley searching for the Glen Terrace trailer park. You don't know where it is, do you?"

"Shit. She's dead?" He too is in shock. It doesn't seem real; doesn't seem possible.

"I'm sorry, maybe I should have called you before. I'm really upset . . . I guess I'll give up. Trish said she didn't *need* me to come. They aren't expecting me or anything. You on your way home?"

"Yeah, but I'm coming that way. Keep your cell on. I'll see if I can find it." He clicks off.

Okay, one more time. I circle out of the empty church parking lot. On my first pass back up Hadley I spot a blacktop drive I hadn't noticed before. There's no sign identifying Glen Terrace, but there's no question, either. As I come over the rise, worn trailers are everywhere. Small gravel lanes run to the left and right in no apparent order.

I stop in the middle of the road, wondering which way to go, then take the first turn to the left. How did I think I was going to find Trish and Dan anyway? I have no clue where Aran lived. Then a dark green Blazer turns down the next street. Is that Dan? I follow behind him.

The Blazer pulls to the side, and a skinny old guy in a T-shirt that says PAPPY on the front steps forward to talk to Dan. The old guy points down the lane. Trish leans out the passenger window, sadly lifting her hand to me, maybe expecting I'd be here.

I park in the shallow ditch and jump out. We fall into each other's arms. I don't want to let go. Dan gets out and hunches against the Blazer, staring at the trailer but not really seeing. When I finally step back and wipe Trish's tears off her pale face, I hug him too. He smells like beer, and I feel his sobs through my chest. Then we follow the old man, who's been watching.

Pappy is fumbling with his keys. "Yeah, the cops was here for quite a while," he says in a raspy voice. "I called 'em. Did you know I was the one that called 'em? Her little girlfriend ran over to my place, pounding on the door, asking for help. I'm the manager, you know. I came right off, and Aran was pretty much gone. I shook her, but it weren't no good, so I went back home and called nine-one-one. She had some foam coming out of her mouth and there were little rectangle pills on the table. Green pills, you know. The cops took them." The skinny old man rattles on, his voice like gravel under the wheels of a pickup. I wish he'd shut up.

The room is surprisingly tidy. There's a worn brown couch against the front wall, a green Formica table on the other side with two chairs, no dirty dishes, a few beer bottles on the kitchen counter, a 1950s lamp. The air smells like mold, or maybe death, I'm not sure. There's a bedroom at each end of the trailer.

"Yeah, around two in the morning they pulled up in a black Caddy SUV. They been here before. Them's the *pushers,* you know. Bad dudes . . ." He puts four beer bottles in the trash. "They were partying. Came in and out of the trailer park two or three times last night. I live on the corner and heard 'em. Nothing new around here." Pappy holds out a small black handbag. "Here's her purse," he says, trying to be helpful.

I would like to be helpful too, but I don't know how. Trish heads for the front bedroom. Dan takes the purse in his big fist and moves that way too, but stops, gazing hopelessly around. He's a tall, handsome, weathered man who's bent over now, like a boxer beaten by the blows of life.

"Is this where she died?" I ask Pappy, pointing to the sofa.

"Yep, right there. The pills were here on the counter. The cops took 'em. Little green *rectangled* pills is what they were . . . Here's a picture of her friends." He hands me a Polaroid. Three handsome young men dressed in baggy pants and long T-shirts stand with their arms around one another, laughing. Were they really the pushers or just some other kids who liked to get high? They don't look too different from Orion and Zen a few years ago.

Dan takes the photo, glances at it, and tosses it back on the table. "Somebody's got a bull's-eye on his back!" he barks and slams the screen door behind him. Trish turns in slow motion, a diver under water.

"Take care of Dan," she says to me, moving toward the back bedroom. I know what she means. Dan has a temper. *Keep him away from Pappy. Don't let him get in a fight.* That's what she means.

"These are my beds," Pappy is saying. "Both of 'em. And my table. There's food in the fridge," he goes on. "And those fans, I better take those." He gathers stuff up.

Trish stands at the open door of the second bedroom. I'm behind her, with one hand on her shoulder. "Dan was here once a few weeks ago," she says. "He came to get Aran when we went to Indiana, but I've never seen it. I had to come."

A narrow cot with a flowered blue quilt is made neatly, with pillows arranged against the wall like a couch. In the corner a floor lamp stands, with a silk paisley scarf draped over the shade. There's a bureau and a closet, a chair. That's all, except one pink high-heeled sandal thrown on the bed.

"This is her room," Trish says to no one. "I can tell. This is *her* room." She turns and I hold my friend while she sobs. I stare back over her shoulder at the lamp, at the paisley scarf. Then we return to the cars with the purse. That's all we take. We leave the pink shoe.

Down in the darkening road, Dan stands by the Blazer, smoking. The tip of his cigarette moves through the dusk. "Thanks for coming," he says to me. "We appreciate it." Trish blows her nose. Then we all turn as a silver 4Runner parks in the lane and Tom gets out. Somehow he's found us. He puts his arms around Trish and gives her a hug. Dan reaches out and they shake hands the way men do, looking into each other's eyes.

"I was supposed to go first," Dan says, wiping his tears. "I thought I would die first . . . I always thought I would die first." Tom nods, understanding. We stand helplessly in the middle of the road. Eyes watch us from the windows of neighboring trailers.

"Do you want us to take you home?" I ask Trish, realizing that Dan is half under the influence and she is half crazy with grief.

"No, we'll be okay. I've got to get home to Melody. The neighbor lady took her." Her eyes are way too tight at the edges. She reaches for the keys, and Dan passively hands them to her, then we all back down the narrow lane. First the 4Runner, then the Blazer, then the Civic. I'm the last one to leave, and Pappy puts out his hand like a traffic cop. I roll down my window.

"I did what I could," the old man announces. "I called nine-one-one right away, but there was that pink foam coming out of her mouth."

"It was probably already too late," I respond.

"There were little green *rectangled* pills on the table."

"You mean capsules? Long capsules?"

"No, regular pills. You got a pen and paper?" Putting the car in park, I reach into my purse, wondering why I'm still here and what difference it makes what the pills look like. Pappy puts down the fans he's carrying, and I watch while he sketches, realizing for the first time that he's been through a traumatic event too and needs to talk about it.

"They were regular pills, not capsules, and they were *rectangled*." He draws a *triangle* about three-eighths of an inch wide and hands the scrap of paper back to me. "The police took the bottle . . ."

"I'm sure you did everything you could. It was a terrible thing."

"It was those pushers to blame. The cops been in here before asking questions. They should have put 'em in jail. She was a sweet little girl."

I nod, then we're quiet.

"Well, I've got to go, Pappy." His gnarled hand rests on the open window. For a second I think of touching it, but Pappy pulls back and gently pats the roof of the Honda two times, then picks up his fans. "See ya," he says, and walks up the hill.

"Yeah, see ya."

ARAN

The Toyota winds slowly up the narrow snake of blacktop. "It's beautiful up here," I say to Tom. "No wonder Trish loves it." We follow the narrow road up Perry Mountain. In the woods graceful white trillium line the forest floor. On either side of the ridge, green pasture falls away revealing a view of more mountains and then of rolling hills toward the west. As usual, we're running late. "Do you even know where Faith Chapel is?"

"They told me it's a mile past Trish's house." Tom's wearing a blue shirt and a tweed sport coat and tie. He doesn't own a regular suit. I wear black slacks and a white silk long-sleeved blouse. This is the best we could do for mourning clothes.

"But do you know where her house *is?*" I get like this when I'm nervous.

Tom gives me a look. "I was here that time we borrowed their power washer. Don't you remember?"

"Oh, yeah." I stare at the envelope in my lap. I stayed up past midnight writing a eulogy for Aran's funeral and I wonder if I'll have the courage to read it. I don't want to cry in front of an audience.

At the top of the ridge is a small stone church with a white spire. It crosses my mind that it would be a romantic spot for a wedding, only Aran will never *have* a wedding. I wonder if this has occurred to Trish too.

A tree-lined gravel drive winds up to the country chapel where pickups and SUVs are parked everywhere among the old oaks. A funeral director in an elegant black suit motions us to the rear of the church, and we find seats on a well-polished pine bench next to Celeste and Abby.

The organist is already playing "Nearer, My God, to Thee," and if I stretch my neck I can just see Trish and Dan in the front pew. They're four feet from the polished oak coffin that holds Aran's beautiful dead body displayed like Snow White. She's wearing a simple light blue dress, but she looks so sad. And no matter how many dwarfs cry for her or how many princes kiss her, she won't ever wake up. Half the people in the congregation are in their late teens, young people Aran went to high school with, probably partied with. A large-breasted soloist stands up and begins "Faith of Our Fathers" in a nasal contralto. I glance again at the envelope.

Tom elbows me. The preacher asks, "Would anyone like to say a few words about the deceased?"

"Are you gonna do it?" Tom whispers. I shake my head no. What was I thinking? I couldn't get halfway through my eulogy without breaking down, not just shedding a tear, but falling apart completely. I open the envelope and read to myself as the congregation begins the last hymn.

The death of Aran has shaken all of us; partly because she
was so young and beautiful and bright, and partly because we

cannot understand it. Somewhere she lost her way. She fell into a place where no one could help her. Not Trish and Dan or her family or her friends or her health-care providers.

When bad things happen I always want to learn something from the situation, maybe something that can prevent a similar circumstance from happening. That's the trouble with Aran's death. I don't know what the lesson is.

All I can say is, we should appreciate each other now, every day, because we don't know how long we or they will be here.

Aran left us her baby girl, Melody, and the many good memories we have of her.

I like to think that she is now an angel guarding other young mothers and babies, holding us all in her love, as we hold her in ours.

I'm ashamed of myself for not being able to stand up and read my eulogy. I tighten my mouth and fold the piece of paper four times. Then the congregation gets up to leave.

We are nearly the last to greet the family on the way out. Trish stands bravely, wearing a slim black dress with a white collar, shaking everyone's hand. Her sandy blond hair is pulled back with a gold clip and she has on small gold hoop earrings. I wonder if she had to go shopping for funeral clothes. I wonder if she took the Valium Tom sent over with Donna and Linda when they brought casseroles to her house.

Dan's eyes are red from crying, his face redder still, and he looks as if he hasn't slept for days. *Life isn't fair,* I think for the hundredth time. The world has tilted too far off balance and I'm not strong enough to right it. I cry only when we file past the coffin and I reach over and touch Aran's blue dress.

Betrayal

At five when Tom calls, I can tell by his voice what kind of day he's had. "I'm on my way home," he says. That's all. Not good. Outside the kitchen window, the crescent moon is already sitting on the edge of the frayed purple sky.

When he opens the front door he doesn't yell out, "Where are you?" or "That soup smells good." I hear his briefcase drop in the hall.

"Hey," I call from my office where I'm answering e-mails. "What's up?" He ambles into the room. His color is off. Something's wrong. "How was your day?" I ask casually. He hates it when I interrogate him.

"Fine," he says. That's all he says.

It isn't until dinner that he comes out and tells me. The office has received another request from a law firm for medical records. I lose my appetite and there's no sound but the scraping of silverware. When he doesn't say anything else, I ask, "What patient? Have I seen her?"

"Elaine Wright. I don't think so. She was that laparoscopy I did a few months back, the one with the nick in her bladder."

"I thought you noticed right away and had it repaired by the urologist."

"I did."

"So why are they suing?"

"We don't know for sure they will. It's just a request for records. I never met her husband but when I made post-op rounds the nurses said he was a pill, a real troublemaker. Elaine seemed fine. I was more worried about a ding on my record for the peer-review committee than a lawsuit. But she never came back for her follow-up appointment."

"You think I should call her?"

"Nah, forget it. It's probably gone too far for that."

I watch the candle flicker on the dining room table, the way it throws shadows on the white walls and high ceilings. Tom's hands lie flat on the tablecloth, his wide hands with the sensitive fingers, his competent surgeon's hands. I don't look in his eyes, afraid of the sadness.

"So who's the lawyer? Is it that same group, McKenzie, Rogers, and whoever?"

"No, some guys from Pittsburgh. Aren't you going to eat your soup?"

·"I'm full." Not true. I'm really just sick. "Did you talk to the urologist? Did the patient have any bad outcome afterward? Did Elaine say anything to him about suing?"

"Patsy, can you stop? This is the reason I don't like telling you things. I don't want to talk about it all the time. I considered not saying anything because you get so wound up. There's nothing to do but wait." He pushes up from the table, throws his napkin in my direction, and heads for his study. Alone, I gaze out at the budding peach trees and beehives below the garden. What other lines of work carry this risk, this kind of threat?

Patients have to sign consents for a reason, and the surgeon has to write down the known complications of the procedures they're consenting to: bleeding, injury, infection. No one is perfect, but apparently some patients think we should be. Whenever the office gets a letter from a law firm, I feel betrayed.

I've never actually been in the courtroom, never actually been sued. It's the *fear* of litigation that gets me. Every day I see twenty patients. Tom sees thirty. No matter how conscientious I am, I could miss something. Every week Tom does eight or ten surgeries. Over 75 percent of ob-gyns have been sued, and soon nurse-midwives and nurse-practitioners will catch up with them. I stare at the darkening sky, almost purple now.

No matter how hard we try, Tom and I will face a lawsuit sooner or later; if not this time, the next.

TRISH

Trish sits eating lunch with me in my office. It's her first day back after two weeks' bereavement leave. Dr. Wilson would have given her more, but she says if she stays home, she feels worse.

"You've lost weight," I say, appraising my friend. Her wine-colored scrub top looks two sizes too big. "Did you get your hair cut?" The soft sandy feathers frame Trish's face.

"Yeah, I went to the mall, to that cheap place. I had to do something before I came back. I'm down fifteen pounds." She fades off. "I'm sick all the time." She puts her cup of yogurt aside. "I can't sleep and my bowels are upset." She reaches for the tissues on the window ledge to wipe away tears. "I just can't believe she's *gone*. I keep waking up and wanting it all to be a bad dream."

"I know what you mean . . ." *How can I?*

"Here's what's really upsetting me today." Trish reaches for an envelope that sticks out of her flowered satchel. "It's the autopsy report. They say the cause of death was intentional, *suicide*. Oh, I feel so bad for her, Patsy, that she was *that sad, that hopeless,* and I wasn't there for her. Did I tell you she called me the night before she died and asked to borrow money? You know what I told her? I said, 'No. Get a job!' And then Dan took the phone and yelled at her too. Told her she should come home and take care of her baby, that she and her so-called friends should get off their asses and quit asking for handouts . . . Now they say she killed herself. That very night, she killed herself."

"But how can they know that, that she killed herself *intentionally?* Does it say it in the report?"

"No, not in the report. That's what the detective told me, what's his name, Lieutenant Saxton, the one that's been handling her case."

"Let me see it." I grab the envelope off Trish's lap, then, realizing I've been abrupt, ask, "I mean, if it's okay? Do you mind if I read it?"

Trish sighs. "No, of course not. See what you think. They say the cause of death was a methadone overdose. The blood level doesn't look that high to me, but she wasn't big. She usually weighed a hundred and twenty-five pounds. They say she weighed a hundred and nineteen pounds afterward . . ."

Tears come to Trish's eyes and to mine. I know that she's seeing the same thing I am. The thin, young dead body of Snow White on a stainless-steel autopsy table in a cold morgue. I touch her hand. It's as cold as a metal slab. Then I skim the report until I get to the summary: *Cause of death: Methadone overdose.* Trish is right. The blood levels weren't that high.

"I don't know," I say. "This could still be accidental. They can't tell from the clinical exam or toxicology report that she did it on purpose. Methadone is a slow-acting narcotic without much euphoria. I don't think it has much of a rush. Maybe Aran took a few pills and didn't feel anything, so she took a few more . . . then more. Maybe she wasn't used to them. After a while she might have just felt drunk and forgot how many she took. Don't you think? Can't you see that?"

Trish wipes her eyes on the sleeve of her scrub top.

"And what about this?" I roll my desk chair closer until our knees touch, wanting to convince her. "If she *meant* to commit suicide, wouldn't she have left a note? See what I mean, Trish?"

Trish nods and takes a big breath, letting her head fall back against the wall. "Maybe you're right. What do *they* know? That Lieutenant Saxton is such a big jerk. 'We got the autopsy report back,' he said over the phone." She imitates him with a nasal twang and a mountain accent. "'You'll probably get one in the mail today. It looks like she killed herself.' That's what he said. Just cold! I believed him, but it doesn't actually *say* suicide in the report. *Aran was a writer.* She left me notes about everything!"

"Yeah, and remember that old guy Pappy," I put in, "at the trailer court. He kept talking about the little green pills." Trish stares at me, puzzled. "You don't remember that?"

"No, I guess I missed it."

I shift in my seat, sure of myself now. "Yeah, he kept telling me, even after you left, that there were little green 'rectangled pills' all over the table and the cops took them. He even drew me a picture." I shake my head, remembering. At the time I didn't get the significance. "The point is, why would Aran stop at just a few pills if she wanted to end her life? She'd take them all, right? Aran's not dumb, she would know that."

Trish puts the lid on her unfinished yogurt and tosses it into the wastebasket under my desk. "You're right. I shouldn't have listened to that cop. What does he know? She would have written us a note. I *know* she would." The small woman stands, stronger now, defending her daughter. Before she opens the door, I catch her by the sleeve and pull her back. We stand like we're slow-dancing and I remember the dream of the waltz. We are resting our battered mother-hearts together.

Another Day on Earth

When someone you love dies, your life starts over. Right then, that moment, nothing is ever the same again. A blue sky, a snowstorm, the taste of cake, the feel of your own skin. Nothing.

I'm thinking about this as I'm coming out of the hardware store, where I've just purchased a cast-iron park bench for Aran's grave site. The clerk, a friend of Zen's from high school, helps me wrangle it into the back of the Toyota. I'm not sure how I'll get it out by myself, but I've been thinking of doing this for weeks.

Trish is now on an antidepressant that I prescribed for her. She's never taken one before, but there's a time and place for everything. It seems to be helping. Dan still can't talk about what happened and sometimes has uncontrollable rages. Their other children are settled back in school, Melody stays with a neighbor during the day, and Trish says she's changed as a mother. I ask her how. I want the secret. Be strict? Be permissive? Give them money when they ask? Never give them money? Keep them at home under lock and key forever? I want to know.

"Tell them you love them. Tell them you love them every day." That's what Trish says.

Today I'm taking the bench up to the cemetery near Faith Chapel. The grave is beautifully situated under a huge spreading maple tree on top of the ridge. It's the kind of spot where a person could sit and contemplate life, could think about God, or hope, which, when you consider it, is the same thing.

At Aran's grave site, I stand for a minute. New blades of grass grow wispy and thin from the fresh mound of earth. Quart jars of white irises sit near a temporary headstone. There's a wind chime, a ceramic butterfly, and a few photographs left by Snow White's teenage girlfriends.

Twenty minutes later, the bench is situated under the maple. The whole operation was harder than I'd imagined, but I'd maneuvered the heavy piece into the spot I wanted and leveled it up by digging holes in the hard dirt with a tire iron. I settle myself on the bench, leaning back to test it. The sturdiness appeals to me, and the graceful feminine scrollwork; a nice tribute to a beautiful girl. Then I slide down onto the grass and rest right next to Aran.

Since my days at the farm, lying on the ground when I'm lost has been healing for me, a way to find my calm center, and I see that to be buried under the soil is not such a bad thing either. If the energy from the earth is healing me, it's healing Aran.

From this angle I stare at the irises on the grave, almost translucent in the slanting afternoon light, and a prayer comes with a breath of wind. "God protect my boys," I whisper.

I know there's nothing in this world that can keep them safe; not me or Tom or God. If it's not drugs, it could be cancer. If not cancer, a car wreck. If not a car wreck, a fall off the porch—and these are the causes of death that take no imagination.

"And God, help me too. Place your hand on me. Settle me for what comes, the joy and the heartache."

A high whistle interrupts my thoughts. It's the cry of a red-tailed hawk circling over the maple. There are churches I could go to. The First Presbyterian downtown in Torrington. The university Lutheran near the hospital. The little Quaker meeting in Delmont. But this is my church, the West Virginia countryside. This is my chapel.

CHAPTER 16

NILA

"He left," Nila starts out.

I don't know what to think. "Who, Doug?" The woman nods. "What do you mean *left*? Left forever or just for a while?"

"Forever. He just couldn't take it. Gibby wouldn't let up. He would call at all hours and threaten, send flowers, beg me to come back. Then Gib started following Doug and calling him at work. The kids were upset, asking me why I didn't go back to Daddy. Tina started throwing temper tantrums. Buddy's teacher called and said he'd gotten into a fight. Tanya's grades were bottoming out.

"Doug wanted me to leave with him, go back to South Dakota or anywhere, but I just couldn't. I had the kids to think about." Nila is crying. Her thin shoulders shake as she sits on the end of the exam table.

I watch from my stool. The bruise and the black eye are gone, but so is her lover. Gibby had gotten his way. "So what's going on? Doug was supporting you. Can you and seven kids make it without him?"

The small woman looks away and shrugs. "Now that Doug's gone, Gibby is starting to mellow out. He gave me some cash and he's coming over to fix things around the house, picking the kids up after school. And he's stopped bringing flowers, thank God." She forces a grin, tight at the corners, the kind of smile that makes a person seem brave. "The house was feeling like a goddamn funeral parlor." We stare at each other.

"Oh, Patsy, I'm so screwed up . . . I don't even know where Doug went. He just packed up and left. It's been almost three weeks. No phone call, no letter. I assume he's gone back to South Dakota, but I checked Information for a new listing and there's no number in Liberty, where we last lived. Maybe he doesn't love me anymore." She wipes a few tears. Nila's not a big crier. "Of course, Marnie, my sister, is thrilled. Now she wants me to go to church with her. Gibby says he's born again and I should be too. He just wants me to be *happy in the Lord,* he says." She raises one eyebrow. Nila is so slim, now only ninety-five pounds, and her face so unlined, it's hard to believe she's had seven children.

"So how are your periods? Are you regular again?"

"Not yet. Those birth control patches really messed me up. I finally had two days of spotting a few weeks ago. That's it, but they'll come back monthly now. You know me. My reproductive system works like a clock. Well, most of the time." Nila shrugs one bony shoulder. I know she refers to her recent miscarriage, her first complication in eight pregnancies, the baby she'd made with Doug and then lost.

"So what can I do for you today, Nila?"

"I still don't feel right. I'm just so *tired.* I'm taking my vitamins every day, but I'm not myself. I was wondering if you could check some more labs. Maybe there's something else wrong." She trails off and stares blankly at the cupboards over the sink.

The woman, a ghost of her old self, cries quietly, this time for real, but then she takes a deep breath, embarrassed. "Don't worry about me, I'll get it together. With seven kids, you don't have time for a breakdown."

"Do you think you might be depressed?" Nila rolls her eyes, round golden brown marbles in her thin, flushed face. "Well, I know you're *depressed,* but I mean enough that you need an antidepressant. Depression can make you tired, make you want to sleep all the time. What with losing the baby and then Doug leaving, it wouldn't be a surprise."

"No, I'm fine. I'll be fine. Maybe I just needed to cry. I'll just get my labs done. Put down every test you can think of. I lose my medical card next week."

I hand the patient the slip.

"I'm sorry I kept you so long," Nila says. "I know this was supposed to be a quick visit. You always have a way of getting me going. A sympathetic ear, I guess. I don't have anyone else to talk to. Not Marnie or Gibby, that's for sure."

"I wish I could do something more," I tell her. "I'll call in a few days when the lab results come in."

We stand at the door. Nila seems so tiny. I could pick her up and carry her out under my arm. Then she straightens her denim jacket, tucks a few strands of loose hair behind each ear, and plods resolutely down the hall. At the corner she turns and raises one wilted hand.

Where, I wonder, *where is the woman that one morning at dawn took off with seven kids in a van?*

Lost

It's not just Nila. I'm still upset over the IRS pocketing our thirty-three thousand dollars. Don, our accountant, has a specialist in his office who's filing petitions on our behalf, and Noelle is persistently working the telephones, but for the immediate future the money's gone, and more is being withheld by Accordia every day. And then there's the threat of Elaine Wright's lawsuit. I can't shake it, this sense that a terrible storm is coming. Tom acts like nothing has happened.

"What's the sense in worrying?" he says when I bring up Elaine's lawyers' request for records. "I did nothing wrong. They probably won't sue me. Most requests for records don't make it to court. If

you worry about every little thing that might happen, you'll be unhappy most of your life."

I sit wrapped in a quilt, looking out over the dark lake, smelling
the new-mown grass and the lilacs, and take a swallow of my sleep
medicine. Until the IRS stole our money and Elaine's lawyers requested her records, I was sleeping through the night at least once
a week.

I think about quitting the practice all the time now and find myself looking through *Homes and Land* magazine for a cheap farm. I
dream of when I was twenty and planted my first peas. How awed
I was to see them sprout. Life was so uncomplicated then, but Tom
won't even discuss it. As far as he's concerned, we'll live in Blue Rock
Estates for the rest of our days. He's a wolf that has pissed around
the perimeter of his territory and he's not budging. Not unless we
go bankrupt.

I could, of course, resign on my own, leave him holding the bag,
but what good would that do? Financially the practice would be in
even worse shape with one less provider, and unless I actually divorced him I'd still be faced with the debts and vicarious worries. If
we continued to live together, I couldn't help asking each day how
the nurse-practitioners' schedules looked, what the checking account held, and if the IRS had coughed up the money they'd taken
from us.

Even if I was able to persuade Tom to move away with me, how
could we sell the practice? What ob-gyn in his right mind would
want to move to West Virginia, where medical-liability insurance
premiums are ninety thousand dollars and up? And where in the
USA are providers protected from frivolous lawsuits? I'm digging
myself into a hole here, but I don't see any way out.

I finish the scotch and stand leaning backward over the porch
rail, which Tom has finally repaired. The smell of apple blossoms
loosens the spring air. There's something comforting about the
night sky, the wide stretch of stars. These are patterns I know,

Orion's Belt, the Seven Sisters, and the Milky Way. They shine over my home here above Hope Lake, over the abandoned communal farm near Spencer, and over the cottage in Canada.

I scan the horizon, from the hills across the lake to the lights of the vehicles on the faraway freeway and back to our drive, but I can't find the North Star anywhere. I step out on the wet grass in my bare feet and pajamas and look over the roof of the house but still can't see it. I'm bewildered, disoriented. If I were a stranger in a strange land, I'd be lost . . . lost with no compass to guide me.

I am lost.

NILA

At 6:30 a.m. my cell phone goes off. What the hell? The office will be open in an hour and a half. Can't they wait? I shake my head and reach for the phone.

"Hi, this is Patsy Harman." I grope for a pencil.

"Sorry to bother you so early. This is Ann at the answering service. Were you out of bed yet?"

"No, Ann. What's up?" I ask without enthusiasm.

"We had a call from a Nila Wilson. She says it's an *emergency* and she needs to talk to you. She said *you*, not Dr. Harman. And she couldn't wait until the office opened at eight. I thought that was strange."

"Did she say what it's about?"

"No. I asked, but she wouldn't tell me. 'I need to talk to Patsy right away' is all she would say. She sounds upset, *very upset*."

"Okay, Ann, that's fine. What's the number?" I write it down, then dial. Tom's side of the bed is empty. He leaves early when he has to be in the OR.

"Hello," a woman softly answers. "Is that you, Patsy?"

"Yeah, Nila. The dispatcher at the *emergency* service said you called." I always put a little emphasis on the word *emergency,* wanting patients to get the idea that this is not a chat line.

"Oh, thanks for answering. I have to see you this morning," a breathless voice starts out. I frown. This is my day off.

"What's up? Is it something Dr. Harman can take care of? Or one of the other nurse-practitioners? I just saw you a few days ago. I wasn't coming in. It's my personal day."

I planned to get my hair cut, go to the mall, buy a new pair of shoes, and go on a bike ride in the middle of the day. This was a new leaf I'd turned over, to take better care of myself.

"No, I really need to see *you*. It's Tilly, my four-year-old. I think Gibby's done something bad to her, real bad." She stops, and it sounds likes she's crying.

"Is she hurt? Isn't this something a pediatrician or the ER should handle?"

"No, this is something for a gynecologist."

Now I'm awake. "What are we talking about, Nila? Are you sure? Where's Tilly now?"

"Asleep. All the kids are asleep, but they'll be waking up soon, so I can't talk long. Can I see you at the office? I'll be bringing Tilly. I want you to examine her."

I hesitate. "Nila, I don't have a lot of experience with pediatric gynecology. There's a specialist at the university. I could call him."

"No, just you. You won't scare her. You're gentle. Tilly won't be afraid if it's you." She has a point; at the university the child would be examined by an attending, accompanied, at the very least, by a resident and a medical student.

"Okay, Nila, can you get there by nine? I'll call the office and tell them that I'll meet you there. Will that work?"

"I have to get the kids on the school bus and find someone to take care of Josh and Danny, but I think I can make it."

"Well, I have a haircut at eleven, so try." I hang up, feeling selfish. The woman's having a crisis and I'm worried about my hair.

TILLY

At 9:15 a.m., I'm staring out the window over my desk at the white quarter moon still high in the morning sky when Abby taps on the door. "Your patient is here. I thought you were off today."

"Yeah, I am. But Nila called this morning and said there was some emergency, so I told her I'd come in. Do you think you or one of the staff from up front could go into the exam room and read to the little girl so I could talk to the mother in private in the conference room?"

I wait at the big table until Nila joins me. She's dressed in blue jeans with a man's brown plaid flannel shirt, way too big. "So what's going on?" I ask, skipping the niceties. Nila sits down and wipes angry tears from her eyes with her sleeve.

"I'm just so *sick,* Patsy. I'm so *furious.* I'm almost sure Gibby has been molesting Tilly, doing stuff to her. I don't want to believe it, but I think it's true. That's why I need you to examine her."

I glance around. Where are the tissues? I must remember to tell the staff that we need tissues in the conference room.

"Nila, I need to know exactly *what* we're talking about and why you suspect Gibby. Is she hurt? Did Tilly tell you something? These are serious accusations."

Nila wipes her flushed face again and tries to take a deep breath. She stares at me, and her large light brown eyes tear over again. There are dark circles under them, and her hair is pulled straight back and held with a rubber band. "For the past few weeks, Tilly has been crying when she goes to the bathroom. I couldn't figure out why. It didn't seem to *hurt* when she urinated, she just didn't want to go in there. I would have to insist because she started wetting her pants again and she's been trained for years."

I cut in. "How old is she?" I'm taking notes in the back of Nila's chart.

"Four. Just turned four. I figured she was going through some kind of phase and I'd just drag her into the bathroom every few hours to keep her from having an accident. I feel so bad now. You know what it's like with a big family. That many kids are kind of a blur. You're just trying to keep them all clean and fed and the home-work done. Tilly has always been a no-fuss child, but lately Gibby's been paying a lot of attention to her, having her over to his house for sleepovers. I never thought anything of it. It gave me more time with the others."

"I still don't get it. What happened that makes you think Gibby has molested her?"

"Last night. Last night, when I was putting Tilly to bed, she was rubbing her tushy. That's what we call it. *Tushy* for girls. *Pee-pee* for boys. And I asked if she hurt down there and she said, 'No, Daddy makes it better.'

"I was freaked. 'What do you mean?' I asked.

"'Daddy does it in the bathroom.' That's what she told me. 'What? What does Daddy do?'

"'Rubs my tushy.' Oh, what does that mean? It can only mean one thing, can't it?" Nila is crying again.

Where are the damned tissues? There should always be tissues in this room!

"And then she says, and this really got me . . ." Nila tries to pull it together. "Then she says, 'Daddy says he has to do it because you're too busy loving Doug.' I almost threw up. Oh, Patsy, has he been doing something to her? He can't be fucking her. She's too lit-tle. Could he have done it to the other girls too? Is it to get back at me because I won't get in bed with him? It's just so perverted. I'll kill him if he did anything to her. I swear I will."

I picture the small blond hairy man with a hard-on sitting naked on the toilet with the pink, naked child on his knee. Doing what? What could he do? Screw her? Finger her? I take a deep breath.

"Okay, Nila, calm down. Maybe it's not as bad as it sounds. Get a hold of yourself. I'll need you to help me. I want to approach this as a routine physical. What did you tell Tilly when you brought her here?"

Nila is wiping her face on her sleeve again, smoothing her light brown hair back into place. I reach over and tuck a loose strand behind her ear. "I just told her that Mommy had a doctor's appointment and she could come with me."

In the exam room Abby sits reading a Dr. Seuss book to Tilly. The small, fair girl is dressed in red elastic-waist pants with a yellow knit top that says PRINCESS. Her white-blond hair is up in a ponytail, and there's a gap like her mom's between her front teeth. She's as cute as a button. A miniature Nila.

"Hi, Tilly. How are you today? Did the nurse read you a book? Thanks, Abby," I say as the nurse leaves the room. Then I get down to business.

"I already checked your mommy. Now it's your turn. My name is Dr. Patsy. It's nice to meet you, Tilly." I lean down and shake the girl's tiny hand. She wears a blue and green beaded bracelet with butterflies. "Why don't you sit up here?" I indicate the exam table. Nila picks her up and puts her where I ask.

I start with the girl's heart and lungs, letting her listen with my stethoscope. Tilly's eyes get big and she smiles. I peer in Tilly's mouth and feel her neck and shoulders, getting the child used to my touch, slowly working my way to her bottom. She's a sturdy little person, well nourished, well cared for.

"Now I need you to lie down and I'll check your belly button. I'll give you a sheet to cover up, so you won't be cold. Mommy can help you take off your pants."

I have no clue what I'm doing. This is definitely not in the nurse-midwifery curriculum, probably not in the ob-gyn's training either. I figure I'll check the girl's vulva and vagina for evidence of trauma. Maybe do cultures for sexually transmitted diseases. I get out the swabs while I'm waiting. If Nila's right, the molestation may have been going on for weeks.

"How old are you, Tilly?"

"Four," the girl answers in her baby voice, lying on her back and kicking off her pants. "I just had a birthday."

"And what's your favorite color?" I'm gently palpating her soft round abdomen.

"Blue, but I like red too."

"My favorite is blue. Now I need to check your tushy. Can you open your legs?" The girl clamps her knees together and rivets her eyes on her mother.

"Do I have to?" she whispers. "I don't want to."

"It's okay, honey. She's a doctor," Nila soothes. We don't use the stirrups. I just have the child lie with her knees open, feet together.

The first thing I notice is the child's red vulva. No bruising. No obvious trauma. No exudate, but redder than usual. "Do you hurt down here, Tilly?" The girl shakes her head no. "Want to play with my stethoscope?" The girl nods her head yes. While she tries to put it in her ears, she relaxes her legs.

I gently part the tiny labia, which are more like skin folds in a four-year-old female. No lesions, I note. Then I take the Q-tip and run it across the opening and in as far as it goes. The child is playing now, trying to listen to her mother's heart as she babbles away. I put K-Y on my gloved pinkie finger and gently lubricate the introitus, the opening of the vagina. Tilly's legs close reflexively but open again as Nila discusses what kind of ice cream they'll get after lunch.

Now I can see the hymen. It's intact but redder and more engorged than most.

"Has anyone else checked you down here, Tilly?" I ask softly.
"Huh?"

"Has anyone touched you down here?"

"Just Daddy, after we take our bath. It makes him feel better to rub me down there, and it doesn't hurt." My eyes meet Nila's. Both our faces are limestone.

"All done," I say. Nila is having a coughing fit in the corner to hide her tears. "You were great, sweetie," I tell the child. "When you get dressed you can pick out some stickers. We keep them in a drawer in the lab for good children. You're the best four-year-old I've seen all week." *Like I've seen more than one.*

I step into the hallway and call Abby. Her dark eyes meet mine with a question, but she takes Tilly down to the lab,

"What kind of stickers do you like? We have horses and kitties and dogs," I hear her say. Tilly wants one of each.

Returning to the exam room, I give myself time by washing my hands at the sink. Nila sits in the guest chair, her legs crossed and the upper one swinging fast. Her small hands open and close into fists.

I roll my stool over. "I can't find any real evidence of trauma. I don't think she's been penetrated." My tone is clinical, like I'm giving report in the hospital, not talking to a mother of a sexually abused child. "The hymenal ring is still present, but it's red. Gibby may have been putting his finger in there, but probably nothing bigger. I've done cultures for STDs. It's all I know to do." I wait for Nila to say something, to ask me questions or cry. Her almost golden eyes are glazed over; she must be picturing the bathroom and her ex-husband naked, fondling her daughter.

"Did you understand me?" I ask. The mother nods once. "I told you it's not my expertise, but I think you're right. I believe her. Tilly said it so calmly, that Gibby has been touching her after her bath. That may be why she hates going into the bathroom. I think you need to see a counselor, and also the cops. I'm going to give you a name and phone number of a social worker. Hanna Westfield knows about these things, and you should also call your lawyer . . . Nila?" The woman's face is so pale. "Are you listening?"

"Oh shit," Nila bursts out. She's twisting the ends of her long flannel shirt as if it's someone's neck. "Oh *shit*, Patsy. What should I do? And him a big *Christian*. What should I do? I'll kill him. I swear." She begins circling the room, then grabs the pillow off the exam table. I'm afraid she's going to swing it into the wall, knock down the picture of the river at Black Water Falls. "What should I do?"

"Nila, stop. You have to get hold of yourself." The patient turns to me, crushing the pillow against her chest. "Nila, I'm *telling* you what to do. You have to see a counselor and call your lawyer. Do you want me to do it for you?" We're both standing in the middle of the exam room now.

"No, I'll do it." Nila moves to the sink and throws cold water on her face. "I'll do it."

"You'll have to report this to child welfare too, and Tilly will need to be interviewed. Under no circumstance can you let Gibby have any of the kids, any of them. *He can't have them.* Do you understand?"

"The son of a bitch will never see them again."

I take a deep breath. "Well, don't do anything rash. Mrs. Westfield, the counselor, will know the procedures. Everything has to be documented. I'll write a detailed note in your chart."

There's a tap at the door, and when I open it little Tilly comes in holding a streamer of stickers longer than she is. "See what they gave me?" she says proudly, holding them up to her mom.

"That's nice," Nila says numbly as she jerks on the child's tiny pink coat with rabbit ears on the hood.

"You'll do what I say? You promise? You'll report it? If you don't, I'll have to."

Nila flashes a look. Her face is a mask with dark holes for eyes. "*I'll do it,*" she says once more.

I reach out to touch her, to give her a hug, but Nila, half dragging little Tilly, shrugs me off and marches out of the exam room, a soldier going into combat.

PENNY

It's Friday afternoon. "Hi, Penny," I say to the bleached blonde who sits on the end of the exam table. She's wearing a low-cut lavender

T-shirt with a sheet over her lower half. Penny's bare feet swing back and forth and I notice a fungus is affecting her toenails but I don't say anything. "What brings you in today? You look great, by the way. I can tell you've stopped picking."

Penny gives me a slow sideways smile and shrugs. "I guess I'm doing pretty good. I haven't picked for weeks. I never thought I could give it up. My family doctor put me on an antidepressant. It helps too." She furrows her brow. "I'm afraid I have a yeast infection again, though."

I stroll over and examine the patient's face, turning it up to the light. Before we did microderm cosmetics I never touched women's faces like this, and I like the intimacy. The pockmarks that previously marred the woman's pale cheeks and chin are fading. Her skin is pink and healthy. I wonder if she looked like this at seventeen when the gynecologist sexually molested her. Probably better.

"I know it's frustrating to keep getting yeast, Penny," I start off after I return from the lab, where I looked at the slide of her discharge. "And I'm going to give you the medication, but I think we may need to give you long-term suppression and test you for diabetes if the infection comes back again. I want you to schedule a follow-up with me in about a week so I can be sure that it's really gone. If it isn't, we'll try something different."

"Yeah," she says. "I'm tired of this."

I clear my throat. "There's one other thing I want to talk to you about." Penny's eyes shift to the floor. "I know you think I'm being overly persistent, but I keep worrying about what happened to you at the university gyn clinic years ago, the way that doctor sexually assaulted you. What if he's out there still preying on young girls?" Penny stares at her hands, opening and closing them. "Wouldn't you want to stop him if you could?" Now the patient's fingers are twitching. She reaches for her face, then bites her knuckles. "I'm sorry. This is upsetting you, isn't it?"

Penny nods. She has tears in her eyes. When she speaks, her voice is so low, almost a growl, I have to move closer to hear. "You have to understand, Patsy. This happened a long time ago. I've forgiven the man. Maybe *you* haven't. It wasn't the worst thing to happen to me. I've got to go." She stands abruptly and pulls on her jeans. She steps into her tennis shoes but doesn't take time to tie them. "I know you're disappointed in me."

"I'm sorry," I repeat. "I didn't mean to make you feel bad. I—"

Penny takes a ragged breath and snatches the prescription out of my hand. "I can't talk about this. Don't you see?" she says frantically. "I really don't want to start picking again!"

"Wait, please. I'm sorry." I reach out for her, but the woman slips by. She twists away and opens the door. Penny runs down the hall past the checkout desk. She doesn't stop. "I'm sorry," I whisper. She doesn't look back. She doesn't even notice her shoelaces flapping.

Water Dream

It's been raining for three days, and the creek at the end of Blue Rock Drive is coming over the banks. Tonight I'm exhausted and fall asleep without effort, barely aware of the steady sound of water pouring over the gutters. In the thin light of dawn I dream again:

Cold floodwater is coming up from the floor, keepsakes and books float around me. I'm searching for babies, dipping down in the brown muddy water. Where are the babies?

In a roar, the walls of the house collapse. I scream for Tom, but he's washed away.

People are crying. Children are screaming but I can't save them. I'm swallowing water, swept away in the current. Then I remember my boys. Where are my boys? My small boys! Frantically I scan for their little blond heads, hoping to see them bobbing along in the muddy river.

They're gone.

❊   ❊   ❊

I open my eyes, my skin wet, the sheets damp. At first I just think it's a hot flash, but then I remember. In the gray light of morning, I replay the dream of grief and remorse and shake the sleep from my head. *Mica and Orion and Zen are men now.* They would be saving the babies.

I am moved by this insight and lie next to my snoring husband, seeing my now adult children, as steady and calm as their father, leading rescue parties, risking their own lives, working through the night, selfless and brave.

They may or may not have gainful employment. They may or may not have a sense of their own life directions, but they would be first at the disaster site. Mica would be organizing a relief crew. Zen would be building dikes to hold back the river. Orion would be out in a rowboat searching for survivors.

It's 4:30 a.m. Through the open porch door, I hear the sound of rain everywhere, still pouring off the roof, off the leaves, off every exposed living thing. I pull a chair up to the window in the dim light and sit thinking about my kids until dawn. Then the rain hits again, harder, slanting under the eaves.

Break in the Weather

Noelle stands in the door to my office. There's a stack of charts on my desk a foot high, and two patients waiting in the exam rooms. I glance over my shoulder at her, but keep signing off labs.

"What?" I don't like being rude but am not in the mood for chitchat. "If it's more bad news, I don't want it."

Noelle doesn't say anything, just dances from foot to foot.

"Okay." I swivel in my desk chair, stretching my back. "Sorry. You need something? I'm just way behind."

Our billing specialist is grinning from ear to ear, her face shining like Hope Lake when the sun breaks through the storm clouds.

"What?" I ask again, a smile flickering on my face. "Is it some kind of joke? Are you and Linda up to something?" Her joy is contagious.

"We're going to get it back!"

"What?" I'm still clueless.

"The thirty-three thousand dollars!"

"Come on, Don Collins said it was very complicated, very difficult, that it would take months, maybe years, if we even *ever* got it back. He said we might have to write our congressman or get a lawyer. I haven't talked to him lately, but he told me his partner, a tax specialist, was working on it."

Noelle does a little victory jig and turns around. "You can pat me on the back."

I shake my head quizzically, patting her. "I don't get it."

"I was talking on the telephone to a supervisor at the main Accordia Medicaid office today." Noelle perches on the edge of the guest chair. "And I pointed out that they've been sitting on thousands of dollars of our payments for months. Miss Hooper, she pulled our file on the computer and said, 'This isn't right.' Well, we knew that!

"I stayed on the phone for twenty minutes while she looked through the account. She said there were records on us about a mile long but there had been so many people involved at the IRS that the attachment of our funds had never been challenged. She said she'll get us a check for the Medicaid portion, about twenty thousand, by next week, and she'll notify PEIA and the other state payers. Maybe a week, she said, maybe two, we'll get a check."

I want to stand up and hug Noelle, swing her slender body up to the ceiling, but Noelle is not a hugger. She's told me before, she needs *her personal space.* I want to run down the halls shouting, throw open the exam room doors, shocking the patients who are sitting on the tables in their thin blue cotton gowns. I want to shout, *Noelle found our money. She's gonna get it back!*

Instead I say, gratefully, "Thank you, Noelle. Thank you." I look into her shining blue eyes. "You are my hero!"

At dinner with Tom, I save the news for dessert, a treat I picked up at Shop 'n Save for the occasion, Ben & Jerry's. We're eating on the porch, the sun sinking behind the black silhouette of trees against a pink magnolia sky. "A toast," I say, holding out my first spoonful of Cherry Garcia. We clink silverware. Tom looks at me, puzzled.

"Noelle talked to someone at the Accordia office today and they're going to release our money next week. I don't know how she found this woman. She just kept persistently calling. This afternoon she was reviewing unpaid patient accounts on the phone with a representative and she mentioned our problem, told the woman, this Miss Hooper, our IRS story. The lady looked at our computer file and says she is going to put it right. Can you believe that? They are going to send us a check."

"That's great," Tom says, smiling. He isn't the type to get up and dance. He takes another bite of ice cream. "Don't forget, Don had his accountant working on it too."

"Yeah, I'm sure they were filing petitions and sending letters on our behalf, but he wasn't that optimistic. Noelle was persistently on the phone with *everyone*, secretary and supervisor, at Medicaid. When we get the money, I'm going to send flowers to everyone: Noelle, the lady at Accordia, and Don's office too. What do you think?"

Tom scrapes out his ice cream bowl, smiling. "Yeah, send something big. All three of them."

NILA

Going through a pile of labs at the end of the day, I come to Nila's and wonder briefly if she's called the counselor. There's a computer-generated lab report clipped to the front of her chart. All the results are normal but one. I don't even remember requesting the serum pregnancy test on the requisition but I'd checked everything else having anything to do with fatigue. No doubt about it. It's positive. Nila is pregnant again.

How could this be? Doug's been gone, what, a month? It must be his baby. I flip open the chart. There were two weeks when Nila was bleeding and she stopped the birth control patches. Maybe then? I shake my head and try twice to call her, staring out the window at the rain. When there's no answer, I leave a message. "Nila, it's Patsy at the gyn office. I have some lab results for you. Can you return my call at your earliest convenience?"

❋   ❋   ❋

At 11:15 p.m. my cell phone goes off. Tom and I are snuggled in bed watching a video. We both groan. I'm on call for emergencies. "Turn it down, will you?" I whisper. "Hello?" I'm expecting the answering service. Patients aren't supposed to have my personal number. "Hello," I say again. It's still hard to hear and I carry the phone into the living room.

"Patsy?" a woman's breathless voice asks.

"Yes, this is Patsy Harman. Who *is* this?"

"It's Nila. I'm sorry to get you on your cell at home, but I still had the number saved on mine from when you answered my page the other morning."

"Yeah, what's up, Nila?" I shift the receiver to my other ear and sink down on the couch, waving Tom through the doorway to go on with the movie. "Did you get my message from the office?"

"About the lab tests?"

"Yeah, I've got your results."

"Don't worry about that. I'm okay. *I found Doug.* I found him! I'm going back to South Dakota. I'm so happy!" she bubbles out.

Then her voice drops four notes. "But I have to get out of town fast. Gibby is going crazy that I won't let him see the kids. Buddy, my nine-year-old, says his dad has a gun."

"What do you mean, a gun? Is Gibby after you? What kind of gun?"

"I don't know the type. What does it matter? Buddy just told me his dad bought a gun. Gibby was bragging about it when he talked to him on the phone. Doug wants to come get me from South Dakota, but I can't wait. We've got to get out of town. We're leaving Torrington tonight." Nila hesitates.

"Tonight?" I say, wondering why she's calling me about this. "But it's so late and raining so hard . . ."

"Well, you can say no if you have to, but I need to ask you a favor. It's a big one."

"What? What can I do?"

"I have to get some cash. I feel real bad asking and I *swear* I'll pay you back, but we have to get out of here and there's no one else. I'm not waiting around until something terrible happens. Can I borrow a hundred dollars?" She stops abruptly.

"You need money for gas?"

"Yeah, Doug's good for it. He's working at the propane plant in Sioux City."

I shake my head and draw in a breath. "This is crazy. What about your furniture, all your household things? You can't just split." Tom has turned off the video and come into the living room. He leans against the doorway in his tie-dyed T-shirt and plaid boxers, listening. He can tell it's some kind of crisis. "Nila, hold on, I have another call coming in. Stay right there." This is a lie, but I put her on hold.

"What's going on?"

"It's Nila." Tom knows the story of the patient's earlier road trip west with seven kids in a van, the subsequent return to Torrington pregnant, the late miscarriage, and the sexual abuse of little Tilly by her father. "She's found Doug, her lover, and she's going back to South Dakota with all the kids. She sounds desperate and says she has to leave tonight because she just found out that her ex-husband purchased a gun. She sounds *desperate,* thinks he's coming after her. She wants to borrow a hundred dollars. Do we have any cash?"

Tom frowns. "I guess we could get some at the money machine at Quik Mart, but this is a little over the top, isn't it? Lending money to a patient. We'll probably never get it back."

"No, *we will.* I know it sounds like a lot. But she says Doug is working at a propane plant. She says he's good for it."

"So when does she need it?"

"Right now."

Tom shrugs. "It's just a hundred dollars, consider it a donation to the Rape and Domestic Violence Shelter. One less victim."

I smile and kiss him on his unshaved cheek. I could have done it without his approval, but his support means a lot.

The cell phone is ringing. "Patsy. Are you still there? I thought I got cut off." It's Nila.

"No, I'm still here. Okay, where do you want me to meet you? I'll have to stop at a money machine."

"We're loading up now. You know where I live? Out on Weimer Road? Could you meet me by the Dairy Queen at exit ten on the freeway? I'll be driving a big blue Chevy van."

"By the Dairy Queen at the Pinewood exit?" I'm trying to picture the spot and don't want to end up sitting all night at the wrong place.

"Yeah."

"What time?"

"Half an hour."

"You really think Gibby is coming after you tonight, Nila? It's so late to start a cross-country trip. Is the van in good shape?"

"No. It's a bucket of bolts, but I gotta go. We'll be okay. I've already told the kids we're leaving. They're scrambling around to get ready. I just have a bad feeling about Gibby. The son of a bitch bought the gun this afternoon, then called Buddy to brag about it, made a big deal. He knew Buddy would tell me. You know how he's been lately. I'm not taking chances."

"Can you really get to Pinewood in thirty minutes?"

"I'll be there. The kids are loading a few changes of clothes right now."

"Okay, see you there." I check my watch. "I'll see you at midnight."

As I pull on my jeans, Tom comes into the bathroom with his worn leather wallet. "What kind of a vehicle is she driving? She's got all those kids. We'd better give her more. One hundred dollars in gas won't get far." He peels off four twenties. "Get more at the ATM."

❋   ❋   ❋

"I just need the money machine for a second," I yell to the young man who's locking the door to the convenience store. "Please, this is an emergency." The pimple-faced guy in the red Quik Mart shirt backs away from the door and glances at the clock above the register, then jerks his head that I can enter. Inside, I'm so nervous I forget my password at the money machine. *Glaze, Potter, Photo* . . . I can't remember.

"We're closing in five minutes," the guy says, lighting a cigarette and blowing it out the door.

"Okay, okay. I'll be out of here." *Daisy.* That's it. I punch the letters in.

The machine coughs up three hundred dollars. "Thanks a million. Is your cash register still turned on?"

He sighs resignedly and nods, so I run up and down the aisles grabbing cookies and juice boxes. I throw him a ten as I run to the car. "Keep the change." Nothing like a little health food for a road trip. There's no traffic this time of night between Hope Lake and exit 10. If I push I should be there by midnight.

Twenty minutes later, sitting in the dark in the gravel lot at the

Dairy Queen, I begin to wonder: *Do I have the right spot? She did say exit 10, didn't she?* I'm thinking of calling Tom on my cell when a dark van pulls up and someone rolls down the window.

A towheaded school-age boy leans out. "Are you Mrs. Harman?"

Is that a *blue* van? In the dark I can't tell. "Yeah, is that Nila?" I know it is but worry that somehow I'll be the victim of a clever ruse. This could be some *other* van full of children trying to get my money. I jump out of the Civic with the roll of bills. "Hey."

Nila, her hair pulled up in a sandy ponytail, wears her worn jean jacket. She bounces out of the vehicle and runs to my side. "Oh, Patsy. Thank you so much." I hand her the money and she smooths it out flat. "This is more than a hundred dollars." She counts it. "This is three hundred and eighty dollars."

"Tom thought you'd need more."

Nila lights the night with a smile and hugs me. Her head comes just under my chin and I hold her too long, knowing I may never see her again and wanting to give her my last bit of strength. By the red neon light of the Dairy Queen sign, her face looks flushed.

"Well, I gotta get going." She stares down the road, looking for Gibby. "I want to make it to Columbus tonight." Then she ducks out of my embrace, trots to the van, and gets in. "Don't worry. I'll get this back to you." She holds up the money balled in her fist. "And don't *ever* tell Gibby where I've gone." Nila waves again and spins out in the gravel.

"Wait!" I yell after her. "Wait! I forgot." I run across the parking lot, and when Nila stops I lean into the driver's-side window. Seven serious children of all sizes stare back at me. Three are strapped in car seats. "I got your labs back. I found out why you're so tired. You're pregnant again. You and Doug are pregnant with a new baby!"

Nila grins. "I figured."

"You figured?"

"Yeah, you know how I am." She beams. "My nipples are sore,

and no period. I was a little sick to my stomach yesterday." She touches my cheek with the tips of her fingers. "I'll write . . . You're a peach."

As the red lights of the van fade away I hear geese overhead in the dark wet sky. Geese going north again, going home to breed. I get back in my Civic and stare at the bag of food that I'd purchased for Nila and the kids.

When I walk into the bedroom, Tom's watching a nature show on PBS about global warming. "No dieting tonight." I toss the bag of chocolate chip cookies on the bed and go to the fridge for two glasses of milk.

Almost Heaven

I'm driving a vanload of artwork across West Virginia to Athens, Ohio, in the 4Runner. Orion has a show in a gallery in Cincinnati next weekend, and I'm meeting him halfway to trade vehicles. These four-foot-by-five-foot framed prints and drawings have been stored in our basement for months. Our son has nowhere to keep them in his narrow walk-up in the city. Tom offered to come with me but was pleased when I said I'd make the run alone. He gets so little time at home lately. This will give him a chance to work in his pottery studio. My only worry is that with no one to keep me company, I'll fall asleep at the wheel.

I pick up the freeway at Clarksburg and take Route 50 toward Parkersburg, passing the exits for West Union, Salem, Cairo, and North Bend State Park. This isn't the scenic route, but all of West Virginia is scenic. Along the freeway the creeks are swollen from days of rain. Last week a woman and her grandson were killed near here when their trailer was swept away in a flash flood. I pass signs for Raccoon Run, Ten Mile Creek, and Dark Hollow.

Thirty miles into Ohio, I miss the turnoff to Athens, home of Ohio University. This is where Orion got his bachelor of fine arts, but I haven't been here in over two years. I circle down State Street back to Bob Evans, a chain restaurant with comfort food. Here, Orion and I meet for dinner and to trade vehicles for a few weeks, his small Honda for the 4Runner loaded with artwork.

I look across the table at him. "So how are you?"

He's shaved his long goatee and I can now see the cleft in his chin, just like Tom's. His eyes are like Tom's too, the warm green of summer fields. He shrugs as he cuts up his steak. "I met a new girl," my middle son says, wiping his mouth.

This sounds positive. "Yeah?"

With my boys, if I appear overly interested they'll clam up, so I casually stare at the family in the next booth, but all my attention is on Orion. "She someone from the university?"

"No, I met her at the bar where my artist friends hang out on Fridays. She's a nursing student at the community college. Really cute." He smiles and raises his eyebrows. "We hit it off. She has a two-year-old."

I shrug. "Mica was two when I got together with Tom."

We eat for a while, not saying anything. Though physically he so much resembles Tom, inside Orion's like me, intense, dramatic, sensitive.

"Did you ask her out?" I finish my salad and push away my plate. Orion is only half done with his steak. He's the slow eater in the family.

"Yeah, I'm taking her to the zoo on Saturday with her little girl, Lizzy."

We finish eating and stand behind the restaurant, ready to leave. "I got an e-mail from Lucy the other day," Orion says, carefully adjusting his drawings and prints in the back of the 4Runner. "It's been almost two years since she left me. It's funny, I found I wasn't angry at her anymore. She's going out with some sculptor in DC. I didn't even care, just wished her well. It was a good feeling."

We hug in the parking lot. Orion holds me tight against his worn brown leather jacket. "Thanks, Mom," he says and gives me a grin just like his dad's.

Fifty minutes later, back into West Virginia, I once again pass the signs for Dark Hollow, Ten Mile Creek, and Raccoon Run. My eyes are getting heavy. I shake my head and open the window to breathe deeply the scent of honeysuckle and hay. We got the check from Accordia on Friday as Miss Hooper had said we would. I have to remember to order everyone flowers.

Ahead, the full moon rises over the hills, shining golden like a porthole to heaven. I'm getting sleepy again and shake my head. When I turn on the radio a song comes on like the sound track of a movie. It's John Denver.

Country roads, take me home.

ARAN

"Trish? It's Patsy. Can you talk?" I hold the phone under my ear as I sort the mail at the dining room table.. The door to the porch is open and the sound of the peepers comes in with the sweet fragrance of lilacs.

"It's kind of a bad time; what's up? Melody's fussing." I can hear the sound of a wailing baby in the background.

"I know, it's almost nine o'clock, too late for a call, but this can't wait. Can you call me back after you get the kids settled?"

"I don't know, Pats, I'm beat. It's been an exhausting day. I'll probably fall asleep with Melody. Is it important? I mean, could it wait until tomorrow? I'll meet you for lunch."

"Yeah, I guess so, but you might want to hear this tonight. I was going through some of the stories I've been writing and found one about Aran. You know what we were talking about before, about the autopsy and what that cop told you?"

"You mean the detective saying she committed suicide?"

"Yeah."

There's a moment of silence, and I make a face. Maybe this was a bad idea. Finally, Trish sighs resignedly. "Okay, just give me a sec, let me see if Dan can feed Melody. Hold on." The phone clunks down on the table. There's silence on the line and then—

"Okay, I'm back. Let me close the door. I'll do the dishes while we talk."

"No, you better sit down. I found something that Aran said to me a long time ago. Remember that time I asked her about depression? Remember that? When I read this I felt she was speaking right to us."

Trish sighs. "I'm sitting." I hear the scrape of a chair, can picture the sink full of dishes, the smell of meat loaf still in the air.

"Well, it was the visit I had with Aran in the exam room right after she started staying out all night. Remember? I was concerned she had postpartum depression and was soothing herself by getting high or drunk. I told her the story of when I used to live on the farm and had postpartum depression. So, are you ready for this?"

"Yeah, go ahead. I'm sitting." I can tell that she's not. Plates are clinking softly in the background, but I go on.

"Okay, so here's what I wrote. I printed it out. We were in the exam room and I'd just asked her if she ever thought of killing herself, you know, just to escape. And this is what she told me, word for word. I swear, Trish, this is exactly what she said."

I clear my throat, reading Aran's words aloud. "'*No,* I could never do that. I think that this is the life God gave me and even if it hurts right now, everything happens for a purpose. I really believe that. I didn't want to have a baby. I never wanted to be a mom. I don't even like little kids very much. But I got one, for whatever reason. I would never kill myself. *I would never.*'"

There's silence on the other end of the phone, no clinking, no breathing. "Trish? Did you hear that? *She would never kill herself. Never.*"

"Thanks, Patsy." I picture Trish with her eyes closed, her sandy head leaning back on the kitchen wall.

"Are you okay? I'm sorry. Did it make you feel worse? It made me feel better. Her death was an accident. I'm sure of it."

"No, I'm okay. It's good. I'm glad you called. Can I get a copy of that for Dan?"

"Sure. I'll bring one tomorrow . . . I'm really sorry if I made you sad."

"No, it's just that when you read what she said I could hear her voice so clearly, and I miss her so much. Even if she was rotten sometimes, I miss her, and she's never coming back—" A door opens and I can hear Melody crying again. "I got to go now," Trish says, and the line clicks off.

Shit. I'm not sure the call was the right thing to do. Maybe I should have waited. I'm always so impulsive.

I read the passage to myself again, remembering the beautiful teenager.

"I would never kill myself. *I would never.*"

Pestilence

Something is wrong today, I can tell. All morning I've heard my husband sigh. I know that sigh. He's depressed. I watch him as he passes back and forth from his exam rooms to the lab. He's avoiding me.

At noon I tread cautiously into his office, put his bag lunch on the desk, close the door, and flop down in his leather guest chair. "Nila sent a letter that she made it to South Dakota without the car breaking down. She's with Doug again and she sent a check for the whole three hundred and eighty. Something wrong?" I ask Tom, touching his arm. "What's up?"

"It's a letter," he says, meeting my eyes. "Another damn letter."

He hands over an envelope with Community Hospital's return address.

"What is it?" I remove the stationery and contemplate the signature on the bottom: Leonard Noble, MD, Chief of Staff. "What does he want?"

Tom opens his cheese sandwich on whole wheat bread. He inspects the pickle and mayo, closes it, and takes a big bite. He may be low, but it doesn't interfere with his appetite.

"It's a case from four months ago," he says with his mouth full. "The peer-review committee is requesting my rationale for not staging the lymph nodes in a woman with uterine cancer." He talks while he chews, and then swallows. "I was working with Dr. Jamison, doing a hysterectomy on Cybil Reinhart. She had a bad Pap test, cancer in situ." He takes another big bite. "When we opened the patient and went to take out the uterus, it was all mush, obviously full of cancer. We *could have* staged her lymph nodes, assessed the invasion of cancer, but it wasn't necessary." He sighs again. "She'll *still* get both chemotherapy and radiation."

"So why does Noble need to talk to you?" My paranoia is running wild. "Maybe the committee's going to restrict your privileges? Did the patient ever come back for a post-op? Is she okay?" I'm pacing around the room like a trapped lioness. "Maybe she's seen a lawyer. I'll call her, see how she's doing, feel her out."

I should stop, but I can't. "You call Dr. Jamison and see if he got a letter from peer-review too—"

"Stop, Patsy. That's why I don't tell you about these things."

"What things? Are there more?"

"Yeah," he snaps. He's being mean now, and throws it out. "Mrs. Teresi, the neurologist's wife with post-op complications, failed to show up for her follow-up appointment today. When I had Sherry call her, all Dottie Teresi would say is she's never coming back to our practice. She's seeing a gynecologist in Pittsburgh from now on."

Something splits open in me. Something purulent and rotten,

like a boil that's been festering just under the skin. "Shit, *she's* going to sue! Remember, I told you. I *told* you this would happen."

"Do you want the rest of that?" Tom asks, nodding toward my lunch.

"How can you eat?" I shove my cheese sandwich at him and it spills down his front. We both stare at the dime-size gob of mayonnaise sliding down his favorite silk Beatles tie.

"Patsy, get out of here." Tom jumps from his chair, wiping himself. "I don't want your help, and I don't want to be near you. You're crazy when you get like this. I'm her physician. I'll take care of it!"

He's backing me toward the door. My husband isn't a big man, but he's mostly muscle. He hasn't touched me, but there's threat in his voice. When Tom Harman's mad, you don't want to be there.

Still, I'm the one with no self-control. If I had something to throw right now, I'd do it. I look wildly around the room and, not seeing anything I can get my hands on, pull open the door, planning to slam it in his face. Sherry, Tom's nurse, stands just outside.

"Your first afternoon patient is ready in room one," she says formally and abruptly hands me the chart.

KAZ

Kaz frowns as I'm palpating his hairy abdomen. "Do you think Dr. Harman would do a hysterectomy on me?" I pull down the thin blue cotton exam gown to cover his masculine belly. At this moment the mere mention of Tom Harman's name enrages me and I don't give a damn what Dr. Harman would or wouldn't do, but I take a deep breath to calm myself and answer professionally.

"I imagine he would. The trouble is, your insurance won't cover it. I mean, what would we use for a medical necessity? There's no bleeding or pain."

"Yeah, I know, I just wondered."

I turn to wash my hands and hold out the tissues. The checkup over, Kaz pushes up to sit on the end of the exam table. "I'm thinking of saving my money and paying for it myself. Someday, I'd like to stop having these Pap tests." He runs his hands over his hairy thighs.

I'm vaguely uncomfortable, not used to sitting alone with a naked man in the exam room. There's something disorienting about his being here in this safe feminine haven. Kaz has no womanly contours. His body is muscular and hairy. Still, he has a vagina, uterus, and ovaries and has to be examined, like the rest of us.

"You seem a little down today, Kaz," I project.

"I don't know why. My job is going well except for the bathroom thing. I ignored their edict and so far no one has had the guts to challenge me. I've stopped looking over my shoulder expecting someone to come up and say, 'Aren't you the Kasmar Layton who used to be a woman?' It's not like I'm one of the good old boys, but the harassment has nearly stopped. It's been a week since I got a weird letter. The thing is, I'm going home for the first time next week."

"What's wrong with that? Are you worried how your family will react?"

"I guess." Kaz sits with his arms folded across his almost flat chest. He still has small breasts but wears a breast binder when he's dressed.

"I thought they knew all about your transformation a long time ago."

"Well, yeah, theoretically. But *seeing* me is going to be different than *hearing* about it. Anyway, I only told my dad about the change. I assume he's talked to the rest of the family, but I'm not sure. And there will be neighbors, people I've known my whole life." He takes a deep breath.

"Won't Jerry be with you? Does he even know Jerry?"

"Oh, sure. We've been together for years and she's been home with me lots of times."

"So if she's with you, won't that be a help?"

"Well, yeah, but she can't be there until Saturday. I'm getting there Thursday." Kaz sighs and rubs his face, as if washing off worries.

I change gears. "This transition's harder than you expected, isn't it?"

"Just harder in *ways* I didn't expect."

"But you told me your dad is supportive."

"Yeah, he's been one of my main boosters all along. He's eighty-three years old, you know . . . and he's been sending me some of his old clothes. I guess he's always wanted a son." Kaz indicates the khakis and the blue flannel shirt on the chair. "He's really cool. He told me he always *knew* I wasn't like other females." Kaz laughs, cheering up. "Maybe he assumes *anyone* would want to become a man if they had the *balls* for it."

"Well, you seem to," I say, giving him a big hug.

"You're right," Kaz says, straightening his back. "I've got the balls for it . . . I'll be okay. And if they don't love me as *I am,* I say fuck 'em. Right?"

I snort a short laugh. "Right. You're the prodigal son. They've got to love you."

Flight and Forgiveness

All afternoon I go in and out of the exam rooms, clamping my jaw until my head aches. I make nice with the patients but speak to no one else. For a moment back in the exam room, I thought of confessing to Kaz. *You know, buddy,* I would have confided, *things aren't what they seem here. The practice is barely solvent. We have patients who are going to sue us. Peer-review is investigating my husband. My marriage is falling apart, and I can't stand the man who once was the love of my life.* But I say nothing.

All afternoon the staff are walking on eggshells, and Tom and I stay as far from each other as possible. I avoid cutting through the lab and stick to my side of the clinic. No one asks what's going on, but these women aren't dumb. It's like eating dinner with your family just after your mother has a major meltdown and runs away from the table to slam the bedroom door. After that, it's all "please" and "thank you," the scrape of knives on plates, and the rest is silence. As soon as my last patient's annual exam is finished, I split.

In the driver's seat of the Civic, I sit slumped, looking across the health center parking lot. It's not just the finances or this new request for medical records. It's not because Mrs. Teresi is dropping Tom as her gynecologist. The incessant worries of the practice have hollowed me out until whatever was left of my love for my husband and my love for my patients has withered and died, like pea vines in the autumn garden. The next wind that comes along, the plants will be knocked off their trellis. Any wind. It doesn't have to be a gale.

This one minor threat and I've lost my mind, lost my faith about everything! The security guard walks slowly between the parked vehicles and waves. I wave back, just barely lifting my hand off the steering wheel.

I'm thinking of running away again. Tom will be at the med exec meeting tonight. I could really do it. I did it before. In twenty minutes I could be in Blue Rock Estates; in another hour, packed. If I left now, I would never have to see Tom Harman again, never have to worry about getting sued, the shrinking insurance reimbursements, or the debts of the practice.

Tired of fuming, I open the car door, take my bike off Tom's Toyota, which is parked two slots down, and struggle it into my trunk. Then I drive aimlessly down Clifton and across Pinewood to exit 10 on the freeway, the Dairy Queen where I'd last seen Nila. Here, I order a large hot fudge sundae and fries and enjoy every single bite of sweet, salty sin.

For a minute I think I see Gibby and shrink down behind the

steering wheel, but when the guy turns I see that I'm wrong. Feeling fortified and not a bit guilty, I drive out Weimer Road past Nila's old house and then back into town.

On my way up Hadley, I turn into Glen Terrace, searching for Aran's blue mobile home, but I'm either in the wrong lane or it's been removed. There's a cement pad with pipes protruding where I thought it would be. Somehow I expect to see Pappy, the trailer park manager, walking along the road holding a couple of fans. We could sit on his porch and I'd let it all spill out.

I'll leave him. That's what I'd tell Pappy. *To hell with Tom Harman, Golden Boy Harman, respected by nurses and admired by thousands of patients. Well, most of the patients, if you don't count Mrs. Teresi and, apparently, Cybil Reinhart, who's planning to sue.*

I'll move to the country alone. I could do it. Get a little house at the edge of Milton, become a photographer or open a flower shop. I'm sick of this worry and I'm sick of Tom Harman closing himself off, avoiding problems, telling me over and over that everything will be all right. It's not all right! I back down the narrow lane, barely missing a white pickup truck, and turn toward Torrington.

At Riverside Park I drag out my bike and pull on my bike gloves and nylon jacket. I decide to forget my helmet. Who gives a damn? The air smells like rain again, and there's a line of towering gray clouds building up in the west. From the corner of my eye I see a distant flash of lightning. Unusual, the lightning, this time of year. Then I push off with no particular mission but to ride as far and as fast as I can until dark. To ride off this anger. To ride off this fear. I ratchet the gears down and lean into the wind.

I'm calmer now, concentrating on the rhythm of my breathing, the rhythm of the pedals going around and around. I see dogwoods in bloom, graceful, white four-petaled flowers blowing against the dark foliage, and the sun slanting in under the clouds. There's no birdsong, no voices, but the smell of the rain is still miles away. I'm riding through a green tunnel shut off from the world.

The trail is abandoned, and I like it that way; no jock bikers, wandering college students, or rugrats on tricycles. Good thing. I'd be likely to run them down, the mood that I'm in. I ride hard with my head down, concentrating on speed, imagining I'm in a race with other middle-aged women. The fans cheer me on as I make gains on the female in front of me.

Behind, there's a low, distant rumble. When I look back, mountains of black thunderheads are massing on the horizon, with the sun setting crimson and gold underneath. For a moment, I stop to stare at the spectacle. It's bad weather coming, but a long way off. I ride on past the waterfalls, carved into the stone on the hillside, swollen now and dashing down to the river. I fly past the lumberyard and the boat ramp where the Jefferson spills over the banks. Then the tops of the trees begin to bend. *Maybe the storm's not so far off,* I think, but keep riding.

It just isn't worth it, living this way. Life is too short. I think of Nila and Kaz, changing boldly, living their dreams. I think of Trish and Holly and Rosa, crying in the night for their children, then rising at dawn each day to go on. I ride harder. It's getting dark fast.

Lightning flashes again, this time closer. The whole trail lights up. I count the seconds, "One thousand one, one thousand two, one thousand three—" then thunder cracks. I lower the gears and push harder, struggle forward. The mass of gray storm clouds is gaining on me.

When the rain finally comes, it's a sprinkle at first, but the sky lights up almost purple, and thunder booms at the same time. I've ridden in rain before, but the temperature's dropping fast. Then the storm breaks for real, big drops, almost hail.

I pull under an oak and wipe my face on the back of my bike glove. In the darkness I can't see anything but huge forks of lightning through a sheet of water. The sky flickers like strobe lights, white then red. I'm soaking wet and freezing. I'm exposed near a river in a lightning storm, holding a metal bike, standing under the only tall tree around. This doesn't sound smart. Thunder rolls up through the valley again.

Now lightning is attacking the earth, as in a continuous war zone. Branches fly past like shrapnel. Nothing has hit me, but something will if I don't find shelter. Before me is five miles of trail to the gazebo near the lumberyard, but it's six miles back to town and my Civic, and to get there I'll have to go through the eye of the storm. I make my decision.

Now I'm riding hard directly into the wind with my head low, wishing I'd worn my bike helmet. If this is a cloudburst, I've never seen anything like it. Each time I pass a waterfall, roaring over the path, I think of flash floods. Dead leaves and mud have plugged up the culverts. Water pours like a stream down the bike trail.

Near the boat ramp I narrowly avoid breaking my neck where a tree has blown over in front of me. As I struggle to find a way through the branches, my slacks catch on a branch and rip up to my knee, but this is the least of my worries. There's nowhere to hide, nowhere to go but forward.

Then I'm riding again, riding through the most frightening electrical storm I've ever been exposed to. My life is a mess, and I'm risking it because of a quarrel. Nothing will change by my running away, not my husband or our financial situation. Not the threat of lawsuits, the abuse of women and girls, or the loss of young life to drugs.

A gust of wind almost pushes me over. I pedal harder, trying to stay upright. Then a branch flies by and I fall. I'm sliding down the ravine on my side toward the river. My bike is on top of me and my face in the mud. I scrabble for a foothold, grab at blackberry vines and multi-floral roses, tearing my hands on the thorns. Then I stop. My shoulder is braced against a sapling on the 70-degree slope.

For a minute I just lie there, assessing the damage. My knee hurts like hell and is bleeding, but my four limbs still work. My shoulder sears where it rests against the young maple that broke my slide.

The Jefferson River roars ten feet below me. Thunder growls up the valley again, shaking the earth.

I carefully roll on my back, staring into the strange dark violet sky, and smile. My life is a mess, but no worse than others'. And my marriage? Maybe not perfect. I picture the gob of mayo sliding down Tom's silk Beatles tie. Not perfect.

I am so *hyperreactive,* so quick to respond. Tom is so calm, so *overly* calm, but we fit together. At the first sign of trouble, I go into battle, brandishing words like a sword. He hunkers down to assess the danger, plan a strategy, or wait the enemy out. While I am planning my route of escape, he is steadily moving forward. *Okay*—the words come to me—*I will follow you.* I'm trying to decide if the *you* means Tom Harman or God. If I knew what God was . . . sure, that would be easy.

Tom Harman, a man who trusts; a man whose cup is always half full. Tom Harman, I may not follow you (and if I do, it's unlikely I'll be quiet while doing it), but I will go *with you,* through the exultation of birth, the defeat of death, the humiliation of lawsuits. I will go with you.

I rest, looking up into the black branches laced together across the sky, like our marriage. I smell the dirt and the leaves and the nitrogen released in the air and I'm thinking, *This . . . this rain is holy water.* Holy water. It washes me clean . . . and for a moment I understand forgiveness.

My marriage is a complicated contra dance. When Tom steps forward, I step back. We aren't always graceful. We take turns leading. Sometimes neither of us wants to lead and we flounder, almost fall over, but we catch each other and dance on.

The anger is gone, not just at Tom, but at Dr. Burrows, who left us precipitously; at the lawyers and patients who sue; at the screwed-up accountants, Bob Reed and Rebecca; at the IRS. I lie in the mud, not cold or afraid. The universe is endless, without a center and without an edge. We are all little specks in the cosmos, some of us more damaged than others, most of us trying to do some good on this planet.

The ground beneath me quakes, and when the thunder cracks again, I sit bolt upright, my hair standing on end. I've seen this somewhere on television, and it wasn't a cartoon. When your hair stands on end you are in imminent danger of being struck by lightning. Frightened, I rise, blood dripping down my leg, and pull my bike up the steep slope, amazed at my strength. I climb on again and push forward into the storm.

It may be the ozone, but I'm feeling great. Even the gash on my leg doesn't hurt. My troubles, like the lightning, strike before and behind me, but it doesn't matter. I'm exultant, dancing on a ridge in the moonlight, swimming naked in the lake by starlight. I'm riding through the worst storm I've ever been in, by no light.

I could be struck dead tonight, but it doesn't matter. The lightning flashes again. The thunder cracks at the same instant, and for a minute I'm sightless. I tip my head back into the rain and I don't stop laughing.

I keep riding, blind, going on faith that the trail is still there.

This book is dedicated to my patients, and I thank them for their resilience, their courage, and their willingness to share.

I thank too my early readers, who assured me that these tales needed to be told; my many midwife colleagues for inspiration; my staff and coworkers who make each workday fun; my writing consultant, Dorothy Wall, who encouraged me to make my words sing; my agent, Barbara Braun, and her team for their endless enthusiasm; my editor, Helene Atwan, for her faith in the project and firm yet gentle suggestions; and the wonderful, hard-working professionals at Beacon Press who showed me that writing the memoir is just the beginning of making a book.

I want also to thank my family for allowing me to tell our story. Mica, Orion, Zen, and Tom, my husband and partner, who is the bravest, steadiest, most optimistic man I know—my metronome.

There's a debate going on about the state of health care in the United States. Everyone agrees the system is in crisis. Meanwhile, health-care providers, physicians, nurses, nurse-midwives, nurse-practitioners, and physician's assistants—along with their loyal staff—soldier on. To those who devote their lives to healing, let us all give thanks.

And finally to you, dear reader, a reminder: In the darkest hour of the night, as you walk the floors with troubles on your heart, remember, you are not alone.